THE
SPOONIE
SURVIVAL GUIDE

JODIE K RANU

GREEN TREE
LONDON · OXFORD · NEW YORK · NEW DELHI · SYDNEY

GREEN TREE
Bloomsbury Publishing Plc
50 Bedford Square, London, WC1B 3DP, UK
Bloomsbury Publishing Ireland Limited,
29 Earlsfort Terrace, Dublin 2, D02 AY28, Ireland

BLOOMSBURY, GREEN TREE and the Green Tree logo
are trademarks of Bloomsbury Publishing Plc

First published in Great Britain 2026

Copyright © Jodie K Ranu 2026

Jodie K Ranu has asserted her right under the Copyright,
Designs and Patents Act, 1988, to be identified as Author of this work.

Every reasonable effort has been made to trace copyright holders of material reproduced
in this book, but if any have been inadvertently overlooked the publishers would be glad to
hear from them.

For legal purposes the Acknowledgements on p. 221 constitute
an extension of this copyright page.

All rights reserved. No part of this publication may be: i) reproduced or transmitted in
any form, electronic or mechanical, including photocopying, recording or by means of
any information storage or retrieval system without prior permission in writing from the
publishers; or ii) used or reproduced in any way for the training, development or operation
of artificial intelligence (AI) technologies, including generative AI technologies. The rights
holders expressly reserve this publication from the text and data mining exception as per
Article 4(3) of the Digital Single Market Directive (EU) 2019/790

Bloomsbury Publishing Plc does not have any control over, or responsibility for,
any third-party websites referred to or in this book. All internet addresses given in this
book were correct at the time of going to press. The author and publisher regret any
inconvenience caused if addresses have changed or sites have ceased to exist but can
accept no responsibility for any such changes.

A catalogue record for this book is available from the British Library.
Library of Congress Cataloguing-in-Publication data has been applied for.

ISBN: PB: 978-1-3994-1150-9; eBook: 978-1-3994-1151-6; ePDF: 978-1-3994-1153-0

2 4 6 8 10 9 7 5 3 1

Spoon graphic: Anna Morrison

Typeset by Lumina Datamatics Ltd
Printed and bound in Great Britain by Clays Ltd, Elcograf S.p.A.

To find out more about our authors and books visit www.bloomsbury.com
and sign up for our newsletters.

For product safety related questions contact productsafety@bloomsbury.com

The information and material contained in this book are for informational purposes only.
No material in this publication is intended to be a substitute for professional medical
advice, diagnosis or treatment. Always seek the advice of your GP or other qualified
health care professional with any questions you may have regarding a medical condition,
including mental health concerns, or treatment and before undertaking a new healthcare
regime, and never disregard professional medical advice or delay in seeking it
because of something you have read in this book.

To my parents, for all of your support and belief in me.

And to the rest of my family, because I'll never hear the end of it if they're not mentioned, too.

Contents

Glossary	vi
Introduction	1
Part One: Physical health	11
1. Living with symptoms	13
2. Living with pain	39
3. Living with fatigue	57
4. The art of pacing yourself	63
Part Two: Mental health	75
1. Depression and anxiety	77
2. Medical gaslighting	89
3. Distancing yourself from unsupportive people	103
4. Imposter syndrome and self-doubt	115
5. Burnout	121
Part Three: Finances	133
1. Loss of income	135
2. Hidden costs of spoonie life	143
3. Education and employment	149
4. Health scams	157
Part Four: Lifestyle	167
1. Social life	169
2. Leaving the house	175
3. Daily living	183
4. Hospital visits and medical admin	211
Conclusion	219
Acknowledgements	221
References	223
Helpful resources	228
Index	229

Glossary

Let's begin our journey together on the same page. To avoid any confusion or misunderstandings, have a quick read of the glossary below, where I have defined a few key terms that will come in handy throughout this book.

Able-bodied	A person who is physically fit and healthy, rather than disabled or diagnosed with a chronic illness, condition or disability.
Ableism	Discrimination in favour of able-bodied people, or against disabled people.
Baseline symptoms	The 'usual' or everyday symptoms a person with a chronic illness or disability experiences. This can fluctuate from time to time and the same people with the same diagnosis can experience vastly different baselines. (See p. 13 for more.)
Brain fog	A symptom of many chronic illnesses, brain fog is a term used to describe symptoms such as poor concentration, limited cognitive function, lack of mental clarity, slow thoughts and memory issues.
Burnout	A state of exhaustion (either physical, mental or both) that can occur due to long-term stress or overexertion. There are several different symptoms associated with burnout, but exhaustion is the most prominent. (See p. 121 for more.)
Chronic pain	Pain lasting longer than three months, and that usually persists longer than the expected recovery time. The pain can be 'on and off' or

	constant. It can also fluctuate in severity, from day to day or even hour to hour.
Condition	A broad term to describe various states of health, including diseases, illnesses and injuries as well as states like pregnancy. It can describe the overall health status of a person, ranging from good to critical.
Disability	A physical or mental condition that limits a person's movements, senses or activities.
Disease	A harmful deviation from the normal state of a person, usually associated with specific signs and symptoms. A general term to describe a wide range of conditions that disrupt someone's vital functions.
Disorder	A functional abnormality or disturbance that affects the body's structure or function. A deviation from normal physiological or psychological function, potentially leading to distress, disability or other impairment.
Dynamic disability	A disability that changes or fluctuates between states. This fluctuation can happen sporadically, daily or within a very short time frame.
Fatigue	Extreme tiredness that is not usually remedied by resting. This is a symptom of many different physical and mental illnesses and conditions.
Flare-up	These are symptoms beyond the baseline of everyday symptoms. A flare-up can occur for a huge number of reasons and represents a marked increase in either the severity or variety of symptoms (or both). (See p. 14 for more.)
Illness	A disease or period of sickness affecting the body or the mind.

Invisible illness	An invisible illness is one whose symptoms are not plainly evident from the outside. Examples include autoimmune diseases such as rheumatoid arthritis or Crohn's disease.
Masking	When someone hides or suppresses certain behaviours, traits or difficulties in order to fit in better.
Medical gaslighting	When a patient feels they are being dismissed by healthcare providers, or their symptoms and concerns are being downplayed. (*See* p. 37 for more.)
Pacing	The act of balancing activity and rest to conserve physical and mental energy and reduce symptoms. This self-management strategy is the main technique for dealing with many chronic illnesses. (*See* p. 46 for more.)
Painsomnia	A term created by patients who have difficulty falling or staying asleep due to their pain.
Pill fatigue/ medication fatigue	A type of burnout surrounding taking medications; a lack of motivation to continue taking your medications. (*See* p. 21 for more.)
Spoon theory	A metaphor for describing the amount of energy a person has. Each spoon is a unit of energy, and each task completed costs a certain number of spoons. Once spoons are spent, they cannot be replaced without adequate rest. (*See* p. 5 for more.)
Spoonie	Related to the spoon theory, a spoonie is someone with a chronic illness, condition and/or disability that limits the amount of energy they have.
Syndrome	A group of symptoms which consistently occur together, or a condition characterised by a set of associated symptoms.

Introduction

Life with a chronic illness, condition or disability is hard. Understatement of the century. Your illness does not care if you have things to do; if you want to socialise with friends or go to the post office or cook a meal. It is the most loyal pet dragon in the world, and will be with you all day, every day, rearing its ugly head when you just want to live a normal life. Unfortunately, 'normal' is relative and your new reality with your chronic illness, condition or disability will look rather different to how it once did. This can be a difficult adjustment to make, and it is usually slow going, but you will adapt in time and create a brand-new version of 'normal'. And that's where I come in – stick with me, and I might be able to make that transition just a little bit easier.

I'm Jodie. I've lived with chronic pain since I was 16, and I'm still not used to it. The pain can still take my breath away and surprise me with its intensity. It likes to keep things interesting, you see. In 2012 I injured my back and it's been downhill ever since. Following the initial incident, I fought for a diagnosis for eight years and was ignored . . . for eight years. I was fobbed off by doctors and other medical professionals and told to lose weight and to exercise instead of being examined and treated. Sound familiar?

After fighting for referrals and finally being listened to – only once I became disabled and began using a walking stick – I was diagnosed with fibromyalgia and lumbar disc degeneration. A double whammy of pain that wouldn't be going anywhere. In order to cope (and vent my many frustrations) I created an Instagram account (@fourmorespoons) to share my experiences, learn more about my conditions and find my fellow 'spoonies' (aka people with chronic illnesses, *see* p. viii).

I am writing this book now as an amalgamation of everything I've learned so far on my chronic illness journey. I am not a doctor in any form and so the information I have gathered and used throughout the book is from my own research, my own experiences, and the experiences of the many spoonies I meet in person and online who also live with chronic illnesses, conditions or disabilities. Medical professionals go to school for years; they learn how the body works and all the technical details of how an illness or disability affects you but, for the most part, they lack the lived experience to provide practical help. As much as your doctor knows about your condition, there is a whole other side to the realities of chronic illness and disability that they likely have no understanding of. Unless they have experienced it themselves, they might not understand how your life is affected on a day-to-day basis. This is why sharing the lived experiences of actual spoonies is so important – why I want to share all my own observations on how to live well as a spoonie and tell you about some of the mistakes I have made in my own chronic illness journey, so you can learn from them and hopefully make your life a little easier.

My goal is to help you survive so that you can go on to thrive. OK, that sounds cheesy, but it's true. I have packed in here as much knowledge, wisdom and insight as I can to help you live your best life as a spoonie. It is my hope that this book will be helpful to you as a survival guide, of sorts, and that it provides clarity and guidance to you as well as to the people in your life who want to understand more.

Is this book for me?

I wrote this book with several different readers in mind.

First, it's for those of you who are new to the spoonie community. If that's you then you can find some much-needed advice here on the day-to-day coping strategies of your new reality and know that you are not alone. There are a lot of people going through all the same things as you, and our combined knowledge has been pooled to write this book to help support you.

Second, it's for those of us who have lived with a chronic illness, condition or disability for some time. If that's you then you can use this book not only as a reminder of the basics (which we often forget along the way), but also as a means of validation as you see your experiences discussed openly, perhaps for the first time. It will also be a helpful reminder that there are plenty of people who know and understand your circumstances, so you're not alone.

Finally, this book is for anyone who loves or cares for a spoonie. It can be difficult to know where to start when your loved one has a chronic illness, condition or disability; it can be hard to understand what they are going through or what will help them. This book can be used as a way to bridge the gap between people in these two very different circumstances.

How to use this book

You can use this book as your one-stop shop for all things chronic illness-related. I have broken everything down into four different parts to cover the four key aspects of life that I believe are most affected by a chronic illness, condition or disability:

1. Physical health
2. Mental health

3. Finances
4. Lifestyle

Each part outlines the different ways in which our lives are affected by a chronic illness, condition or disability, and the tips and advice I can give you to help you live your life in the best way possible.

Feel free to read this book from start to finish, from back to front, or to just skip to the sections you find most relevant right now. If picking and choosing chapters and sections is more helpful to you, and is how you can best spend your energy, then that's how you should proceed.

You'll notice at the end of some sections I have included 'Reflections'. These are questions to think about as you're reading. You could use them as prompts for discussion topics with loved ones and carers or as journal prompts for personal writing. You could even use them as content questions for social media. However you use them, I truly hope you find them helpful and beneficial in your own chronic illness or disability journey.

Throughout the book you will also notice segments called 'Community column' where I add in tips and suggestions from other spoonies in my online community. These words of wisdom are from people just like you, going through similar things as you, whose words are borne of their own lived experiences.

Also dotted throughout the book are 'Key term' highlights where I go into a little more detail about various symptoms, or the technical language being used. These have been added to help break down the jargon, which, although necessary at times, can be quite confusing. For that reason I've also included a glossary on p. vi.

And finally, you'll see little reminders here and there, which are intended to clarify and reinforce the main point I'm making, or to include important additional information.

A note on language

It is important to note that the terminology used in this book is the accepted and most up-to-date language to describe the concepts and ideas discussed at the time of writing. However, as language is an ever-evolving medium, it is likely that in the future some of the terms and turns of phrases may become outdated or change, so I want to acknowledge this. For example, I have used the term 'able-bodied', which is currently the appropriate language to describe a person without a chronic illness, condition or disability.

Furthermore, I would like to acknowledge that not all able-bodied people can do the same things as each other. There are a huge range of factors that go into determining what someone is capable of, such as parenting responsibilities or mental health difficulties, for example. Therefore, I use the term 'able-bodied' mainly to simplify rather than to call out a particular group of people. I am not implying that every able-bodied person has access to the same experiences.

The glossary on p. vi outlines what I mean by 'illness', 'condition' and 'disability', since these are technically different things. To make matters more confusing, some illnesses fall into more than one category. For example, diabetes is both a chronic metabolic disease and a condition. Disability also covers a huge spectrum, from obvious physical differences to invisible disabilities such as neurodivergence or mental health problems. To cover all of these, I will use the phrase 'chronic illness, condition and disability'.

The spoon theory

Throughout this book I'll refer to something called the 'spoon theory'. This is a metaphor created in 2003 by writer Christine Miserandino, and is a means of explaining how much energy is used up doing certain tasks during the day. The spoon theory posits that someone with a chronic illness, condition or disability has a limited number of spoons (units of energy) per day, and that each task that is completed costs a certain number of spoons.

For example, if I wake up with 12 spoons and it costs one spoon to get out of bed, three spoons to take a shower and three more to make and eat breakfast, before my day has really begun I am already down by seven spoons. With my limited energy I would need to carefully consider what I do with the rest of my day. Whereas able-bodied people would be able to quickly recover during the day and gain back spent spoons, someone with a chronic illness, condition or disability has only a set number of spoons to last them the entire day and, once they have been spent, they are gone.

Table 1 The cost of everyday tasks

One spoon	Two spoons	Three spoons	Four spoons
Get out of bed	Get dressed	Cook and eat a meal	Attend a medical appointment
Watch television	Make a phone call	Housework or chores	Exercise (30 minutes)
Take medications	Study	Bathe/personal hygiene	Go to work (including travel)
Scroll online	Read a book	Run errands	Socialise

Table 1 is a little guide to the types of everyday tasks we all must complete and roughly how many spoons they may cost, although of course this will vary from person to person. In fact, a significant aspect of the spoon theory is just how variable it is. When we have a chronic illness, condition or disability there is no way of ensuring that we wake up each day with the same number of spoons. There is also no universal guide as to how many spoons each activity will cost; it is very much dependent on the individual. For example, getting out of bed could cost me one spoon whereas someone else may have more fatigue than me, meaning it could cost them three spoons. The number of spoons a task costs can vary day to day for an individual, too. For example, on one day running errands may cost you three spoons and on another it may rise to six spoons. This wide variation in the number of spoons an activity can cost is due to lots of factors, many of which are outside of your control. This can include the amount of sleep you have had, the weather, your own pain and energy levels as well as if you are experiencing any additional symptoms.

For all these reasons, it can be very easy for someone with a chronic illness, condition or disability to overestimate our energy levels and what we can manage. It's important we take time to reflect on our energy levels constantly throughout each day to ensure we pace ourselves (see pp. 63–73). The spoon theory has grown in popularity as a handy tool for helping us to do just this, and also as a simple and accessible method of explaining to able-bodied people how our energy levels work.

Thanks to the popularity of the theory, over the last decade or so, many in the chronic illness community have affectionately adopted the term 'spoonie' to describe ourselves and many will refer to 'spoons' when discussing current energy levels. Terms such as 'running low on spoons' and 'low-spoon day' are quite common within the chronic illness and disabled community.

Understanding and assessing the number of spoons you have on any given day can be a difficult task and is one you will get better at over time. It will likely take a lot of trial and error and self-reflection to know what types of activity will cost you more spoons and what types of activity have a longer or shorter recovery time. Most of the time you can work off assumptions. When planning your day or week you can make reasonable assumptions about your schedule: if you're spending the entire day walking around at an event on Friday, spoons will be pretty depleted on Saturday. As this is not an exact science, often we must rely more on the art of pacing ourselves (see pp. 63–73) in order to ensure we are not spending more spoons than we have on any given day or week.

Seven essential things you need to know

I have learned a few lessons the hard way throughout my own chronic illness journey. These can be boiled down to seven key things. So, before we kick off, I want to share these with you. Then I invite you to delve deeper into the rest of the book to explore them in more detail:

1. **Put yourself first** (see p. 129). Right, tough love, coming in hot: you need to prioritise your own needs and put your own life jacket on first. Stop being at the beck and call of others and taking care of everybody but yourself. It is not at all healthy to ignore your own needs in favour of someone else's. There is no point trying to take care of those around you if it means you are slowly fading away. That is, simply put, a losing game.

2. **Setting boundaries is crucial** (see p. 126). You need to set physical, psychological and emotional boundaries to help you avoid burnout. At the beginning of your journey, setting these boundaries might be awkward and uncomfortable (especially if you are a people pleaser like me) and you may struggle to enforce them all. However, practice makes perfect, and you need to keep trying until you get it right.

3. **Rest and pace yourself** (see p. 64). This is the only real way to survive with a chronic illness or disability. You may believe that you can stick to your old routines and ways of doing things, but you honestly can't and trying to will lead to problems. Ignore any voices that shame you for pacing and conserving energy (whether they are external or internal) and do what is right for you. The idea that if you slow down or reprioritise you are giving up is wrong, harmful and frankly ableist.

4. **Advocate for yourself** (see p. 96). Be your best advocate and get second and third opinions if you need them. You know your body better than anybody else. If medical professionals try to tell you otherwise, be prepared to fight them. Remember, it is your

right to receive medical treatment and to be heard during your appointments. You are your own priority, always.

5. **'No cure' does not mean 'no improvement'**. Even if your chronic illness or disability has no cure, managing it – and treatments suggested by your medical team – can sometimes lead to improvements, so try to stay open to new ideas and paths you may not think to go down.

6. **Physical health and mental health go hand in hand** (see p. 77). Poor mental health can, and does, impact your physical health. Looking after one can affect the other. You need a good balance of physical and mental health in order to manage your chronic illness, condition or disability.

7. **Finally, be yourself. Unapologetically**. Something I desperately wish I had understood and accepted sooner is this: if people want to judge you for your choices, that's on them. Never let another person's thoughts, opinions or hang-ups dim your light.

Community column

What is the most important lesson you've learned from your chronic illness journey?

'Not everyone is going to understand or care about my situation, so I need to learn ways to keep on going. I don't let anyone stop me or write me off, especially myself. I can be my own biggest supporter or my biggest enemy.' – Bree

'That life isn't supposed to be happiness and rainbows . . . life is an adventure.' – Isabella

'To not take the good days for granted.' – Tasha

'To be easy on ourselves and kind to everyone.' – HP

'Life can still be great. Hard sometimes, but still great.' – Sarah Jane

'I am more than my illness. I am worthy! I am amazing regardless of my illness. I don't owe anyone anything. I must satisfy myself. Celebrate all accomplishments, big or small! Cherish the good days!' – Liyah

1
Physical health

1. Living with symptoms　　　　　　　　　　13
2. Living with pain　　　　　　　　　　　　39
3. Living with fatigue　　　　　　　　　　　57
4. The art of pacing yourself　　　　　　　　63

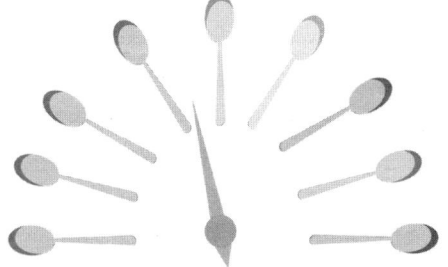

1
Living with symptoms

The physical aspect of living with a chronic illness, condition or disability can be one of the most difficult. The everyday toll on your body caused by constant symptoms is gruelling. Personally, I am in pain every day. Yes, every day, including my birthday, Christmas and today, the day you're reading this.

How to manage your baseline symptoms as part of your regular routine will be covered in more detail in the 'Daily living' chapter (see p. 183). However, here, we'll focus instead on understanding the difference between baseline symptoms and flare-ups, so that you can learn how to identify flare-ups and survive them. If you're new to the community and need help tracking your symptoms, there is advice on this at the end of the chapter (see p. 33).

> ### Baseline symptoms v flare-ups – an overview
> Baseline symptoms are the average symptoms you experience on any given day. The kind of bog-standard things that, while terrible and debilitating for an able-bodied person, you can cope with. Your baseline symptoms are what you have as you live your life in the 'normal' way.

> Flare-ups occur when you experience an increase in the severity or intensity of your regular baseline symptoms. They usually require some extra treatment, such as additional medication, extra rest, or any other intervention required as part of your own individualised treatment plan. A good way to define a flare-up is as an increase in your everyday symptoms that causes you to change your daily life in some way.

Baseline symptoms

Living with baseline symptoms and actively managing them will look different for everybody. Even if you have the exact same diagnosis, treatment plan, medications and lifestyle as another spoonie, it is unlikely that you will both experience the exact same baseline symptoms or the same severity of them. For example, despite both having fibromyalgia, Patient A may experience pain and fatigue as their baseline symptoms, while Patient B experiences more brain fog and pain as their baseline. They have the same conditions and similar symptoms but not the exact same.

It's also important to recognise that your baseline symptoms – and therefore the way you'll need to manage them – can and will change as you move through your chronic illness, condition or disability journey. They may get better or worse throughout your life depending on many factors, including your medications, treatment plan or simply your age.

Managing your baseline symptoms can be difficult, as it requires you to walk the fine line between resting, pacing (see p. 63) and taking medications, while at the same time trying to live your everyday life with as little disruption as possible. When walking this tightrope, try to keep in mind that if you push yourself too far you will end up in a flare-up or burnout (see p. 121), which will disrupt your life even more.

At the start of my own chronic illness journey this was a difficult concept to grasp. I was 16, an age when turning down invitations and getting home early ruined your social life. This meant I frequently attempted to push my own limitations and ended up in flare-ups. For years I attempted to keep up with my peers in a way that should have been easy to do, but for me was a struggle that likely worsened my illnesses and led to lifelong mobility issues.

Actively managing your baseline symptoms can be a full-time job that requires you to pay close attention to your own body at all times. You will need to monitor your medication doses, sleep, activity level, food intake, water intake and more (see p. 34) to see what affects your symptoms. But understanding what works for you and what doesn't is key: it's as much a part of symptom management as taking your medications. For example, knowing that attempting to clean the whole house in one day is going to push you into a flare-up is essential information to have.

So, if you start to feel the increase or worsening of baseline symptoms, stop what you're doing, take stock, assess yourself accurately and acknowledge if you are pushing your limitations too far. Your baseline symptoms are a highly personal and individual part of spoonie life, and it can require lots of self-reflection to identify the difference between your baseline symptoms and a flare-up (see Tracking your symptoms on p. 33). I tell you this not to scare you, but to warn of the dangers of ignoring the signals your body may be giving you. Your baseline symptoms should be respected as the calm before the storm, because if you don't respect your baseline symptoms the flare-up symptoms are usually never far off . . .

Reminder: just because you *can* live with these baseline symptoms does not mean they are not life-altering and serious. Baseline symptoms simply means the daily level of symptoms you deal with on a regular Tuesday. One person's baseline could mean they can work, exercise and live a relatively 'normal' life, whereas someone else's baseline could mean they are housebound and unable to carry out daily tasks unaided.

Flare-ups

A flare-up can be an increase in the severity of your symptoms, such as worse pain than usual or more fatigue than expected. Or a flare-up can be new symptoms altogether. For example, during flare-ups I can often experience migraines on top of my baseline symptoms, as a special little gift from the universe.

During flare-ups try to take stock and identify possible treatments for your additional or new symptoms. Some flare-ups will simply require an extra dose of medication or resting more for a few days to bring you back to baseline. At other times treating a flare-up can be more involved and may require professional help or treatment from a hospital. We'll be looking at common ways to manage flare-ups on p. 22.

In order to effectively treat all your flare-ups, and preferably avoid them, we need to look at some of the main causes.

Common causes of flare-ups

As explained, understanding what might trigger your flare-ups is important, as this will help you avoid and reduce the number you may have in the future.

But, before we start, know that a flare-up is not a failure. Having one (or hundreds) of flare-ups is not some personal or moral shortcoming on your part. Most of the time there is absolutely nothing you can do to stop one. Even if you do everything 'the right way', you can still flare up for seemingly no reason at all.

It has taken me years to stop blaming myself when I'm in a flare-up. It only happened when I realised that this kind of negative self-talk has a huge impact on my mental health, stress and even sleep – all factors that could lead to more flare-ups. In the past, it had become a never-ending cycle of frustration for me. Please try to understand that while it is vital that you learn to correctly manage your illness, condition or disability to the very best of your ability, unfortunately flare-ups are a big part of life for us spoonies, and they are something that you may need to learn to live with.

If you are someone with a chronic illness, condition or disability, then common causes of flare-ups include:

1. Overexertion
2. Poor sleep
3. Poor nutrition
4. Dehydration
5. Weather
6. Medication
7. Stress
8. Poor mental health
9. Sensory issues
10. Acute illness

Reminder: while this is a good list of things that can cause a flare-up it is by no means a complete list. It will thrill you to know that there are plenty of other things that can trigger a flare-up and many of them are not well researched.

1. Overexertion

It should come as no surprise to you that overdoing it one day will likely lead to a flare-up on the next. As spoonies it can be so easy to overextend ourselves and push past our bodies' natural limitations. Personally, even after years with my illness, I still feel a tremendous amount of guilt when I think I'm not being productive enough. This then leads me to push myself too far by doing too much, too fast and causes a flare-up.

If you are feeling like this, bear in mind that by overexerting on one day, you risk being 'less productive' on others. If the fear of being less productive is one you experience, remind yourself that balancing rest and activity will be the only thing that will help you in the long run.

2. Sleep

Ah, the ever-elusive sleep (this is a major cause of flare-ups for me personally). When our bodies are not properly rested, a flare-up is often inevitable. All bodies need adequate rest to function at the optimum level, and as spoonies our bodies are already working harder than other people's. Good quality and quantity of sleep is therefore a necessary requirement to avoid flare-ups, so good sleep hygiene is key.

There are several good sleep habits you can adopt, such as:

- Avoiding screens before bed
- Getting up and going to bed at the same time each day
- Skipping the caffeine (at least six hours before bed)

3. Nutrition

Good nutrition can get overlooked when it comes to symptom management, which is strange, since food is the fuel your body needs to function well. If you forget to charge your phone, you cannot be surprised when it shuts down. It's little surprise, then, that poor dietary habits can lead to increased symptoms over time. Eating some proper meals that are at least somewhat healthy is an effective way to avoid flaring up too often.

If healthy meals are beyond your capabilities, remember that any food is still better than no food at all. Even if that means you rely on takeaways and snacks, eating will always be a better option than skipping meals. And of course some chronic diseases, such as diabetes and Crohn's disease, are hugely impacted by diet, in which case good nutrition is a fundamental part of your treatment plan and needs to be taken very seriously.

When it comes to cooking as a spoonie there are many challenges that we can face on a daily basis, so later in this book I will go through some cooking and eating tips that may help you (see pp. 192–196).

4. Dehydration

Making sure you are drinking enough water throughout the day can often help you avoid an increase in your symptoms. Carrying a water bottle can be useful for this, or you could set a reminder on your phone to drink water at certain times. If you cannot or don't like to drink plain water, drink something else non-caffeinated instead, such as herbal tea, milk, squash or fruit juice – it all counts! Conversely, drinking caffeinated drinks or alcohol has a diuretic effect, which can make you more dehydrated, as well as impacting your sleep.

5. Weather

Many spoonies seem to find that their flare-ups occur slightly more frequently during the colder months and less frequently in warmer climates. As I have a chronic illness related to pain in my joints and muscles, I have definitely found this to be true. However, I have also found that extremely high temperatures can cause their own issues. So, it's kind of a damned if you do, damned if you don't sort of situation, for me at least.

Other types of weather can cause issues, too. For example, spoonies with respiratory conditions might struggle if the air is very dry, or very humid, whereas people with visual impairments or sensitivities might find it especially difficult to navigate when it's foggy, or experience worse eye pain when it's sunny.

A good way to deal with this is making sure you have what you need. For example, in colder months adding a heating pad or hot water bottle to joints when they hurt can ease symptoms. Similarly, adding ice packs in extreme heat will help you keep your cool. I have learned that a happy medium works best, where I am not too cold and not too hot, but it is crucial that you find a system that works for you, your body and your symptoms. Remember, everybody is different, so this may require some trial and error.

6. Medication

Another obvious contender for causing flare-ups is medication. Keep this in mind, as it's common for doctors to need to tweak and adjust your dosages several times before finding a combination that works well for you. Adjustments can also be made due to changes to prescribing guidelines or new medicines being approved for use for your illness, condition or disability. Some medication changes will be good, but others may lead to issues.

Throughout your spoonie journey it is likely that you will experience some form of burnout or pill fatigue, too. Skipping medications or stopping them altogether as a result of this pill fatigue can lead to flare-ups and increased symptoms. It can be difficult to stay on track with a chronic illness, especially as it can feel like there is no end in sight. However, the damage you could do to yourself by skipping medications can last a long time and could make your overall condition worse. As difficult as it may be to do, it is imperative that you continue taking your medications and complying with doctors' orders.

Sometimes missing medications can be outside of your control. Your illness may cause confusion or forgetfulness, and issues such as visual impairment or age-related confusion can lead to patients becoming non-compliant with their medications. In these circumstances staying on track with medications can be difficult, but it is still essential. Use reminders on your phone to ensure you are remembering your medications and ask for help from your pharmacist to ensure the packaging they provide medications in are best suited for your needs, whether that includes large fonts, braille or easy-open caps.

It's also very important to be honest with your medical care team if you are skipping your medications. Whether it is due to pill fatigue or simply forgetting to take them, these missed doses can and do have an overall effect on the management of your chronic illness, condition or disability and so doctors need to know when this is happening. The more information they have, the better your care will be.

> **Key term: pill fatigue**
>
> This occurs when a person loses all motivation to continue with their regularly required medications. It can happen when someone becomes overwhelmed with the number of prescription medications they need to take, and the frequency with which they need to take them. Speaking with your medical care team can ease the burden of pill fatigue, as other interventions may be available, such as transdermal patches rather than pills.
>
> Also known as: medication fatigue or medication burnout.

7. Stress

Another obvious culprit for flare-ups is additional stress, whether that's from work, family, your illness or pretty much anything else. Learning tips for managing stress, like mindfulness, digital detoxes and setting achievable goals in your life, can all help. Additionally, it may be necessary – and a good idea – to seek professional advice for stress management. It's somewhat ironic that stress can cause excess symptoms, and yet having a chronic illness is inherently stressful.

8. Mental health

Changes in your mental health are also a leading cause of flare-ups in spoonies. Our bodies and minds are not separate; they are all one system and having an increase in mental health issues can lead to an increase in physical health issues. For example, depression can lead to symptoms like headaches or additional fatigue, while anxiety can cause digestive issues and insomnia (see p. 77 for more). All of these physical symptoms can trigger an increase in your baseline symptoms.

9. Sensory issues

Sensory issues like sensory overload can lead to things like headaches, mood swings or additional stress, which can all cause a flare-up in your chronic illness, condition or disability. I experience sensory overload fairly regularly and, honestly, it can take a huge toll on my body and leave me feeling wrung out and frazzled. The easiest way I have found to deal with this is to remove myself from triggers (such as crowded or noisy places) and to take the time, in a quiet space, to centre myself.

> **Key term: sensory overload**
>
> This happens when your brain enters a fight, flight or freeze mode as a result of too much input from your five senses, and you become overwhelmed and stressed.

10. Acute illness

Unsurprisingly, adding an acute illness like a cold, flu or stomach bug on top of your chronic illness can make everything worse. If you are in and out of hospital for appointments it is so easy to pick up something like the common cold during the winter and it can really knock you down when you have chronic symptoms at the same time.

So, now that we have discussed the potential causes of your flare-ups, let's take a look at how to manage them if and when they occur.

Common ways to manage flare-ups

Learning to manage your flare-ups is an important skill because they are inevitable throughout your spoonie journey. I have created a list of things you can do, below, once one has begun.

Reminder: this list is made up of things that I have found work well for me and other spoonies in my community, but you may find that other techniques are better for you. So, you can begin with the techniques below but be sure to adapt them to your own circumstances.

To manage a flare-up you could:

1. Rest
2. Get help
3. Take medications
4. Consume food and drink
5. Postpone plans
6. Get comfortable

1. Rest

Let me take a moment to blow your mind. The first tip for managing a flare-up is . . . rest. I know this may seem like a simple first step but be honest here: are you really getting enough rest? If the answer is no, then this may be a problem. When you've got a huge increase in symptoms, attempting to soldier on and keep pushing through can only end badly. It's harmful to overexert yourself in this way and can cause longer-lasting damage and an overall increase in your baseline symptoms for days and weeks to come (or even longer). So, I'll say it again: rest.

2. Get help

The second tip is equally simple: you need to get help during a flare-up. If at all possible, ask your family and friends for assistance with essential tasks in order to take the pressure off yourself. Everyday chores, such as cooking and cleaning, can take up a lot of energy and should be avoided if at all possible during a flare-up.

I know reaching out to others can be difficult. You might feel guilty that you're asking for too much, you feel like a burden, you don't want to disturb anybody else, and about a hundred different other things, but if you need help, ask for it. There is absolutely no shame in it. If your loved ones asked you for help, you'd do it, wouldn't you?

If asking friends and family isn't an option or you simply don't want to, you can look up professional services in your area that may be able to help, as well as local charities with support services. See the resources on p. 228 for more information.

3. Take medications

This is yet another obvious one here – seriously, take your medications! Whether it's your regular medications that you need on a daily basis or extra painkillers to deal with increased symptoms, please take them. There is no need to suffer in agony if there is a straightforward way to ease the problem. Remember, though, if your medications are not helping your flare-ups or working as intended, or if you have concerns about dependency and tolerance, speak to your doctor and medical care team in order to make any medication changes or adjustments that may be required.

4. Consume food and drink

During flare-ups it can be difficult to make and prepare food and drink, and sometimes increased symptoms can lead to a reduced appetite. However, it is important to nourish your body and fuel and hydrate it to keep it going. If cooking is simply too much of a challenging task for you, order takeout food or snack on smaller items instead of skipping meals altogether. If you have special dietary requirements, are a picky eater or prefer to save your money, making portions of cooked food ahead of time and keeping them in the freezer is a good way to ensure you always have a hot meal you can heat up when you are not able to cook. Don't forget to also drink plenty of water (see p. 19). An easy way to do this is keeping a bottle nearby at all times or setting a reminder on your phone.

5. Postpone plans

Wherever possible, postpone or cancel plans during a flare-up. Socialising with friends and family should take a back seat during these times, so that you can prioritise your recovery. This means you may need to miss out on occasions you were really looking forward to; it's not a happy thought, but it is a realistic one. Make your loved ones aware during the planning stage that it may happen, so they are not blindsided if you have to cancel. Missing out on things from time to time is an unfortunate and unfair reality of life as a spoonie, but your health is your top priority.

6. Get comfortable

Wear clothes you find comfortable and that you can relax in during flare-ups, especially if your symptoms include pain, irritation or skin sensitivities. Also, try to relax in a comfortable place doing activities you enjoy and find peaceful, and rest until you are feeling better. Personally, I spend my flare-ups in bed or on the sofa in my pyjamas, watching my comfort shows. Comfort is a subjective thing, so this may look different for you than it does for me.

> ### Community column
>
> Flare-up must-haves:
> - My electric heat pad
> - A comfy blanket (sometimes a lighter weighted blanket)
> - Extra pillows for under my knees and back
> - My two cats for snuggles
>
> – Bec
>
> - Massage gun
> - Compression socks
> - Support braces
> - Noise-cancelling headphones
>
> – Anonymous

Reflections

How could you implement this management strategy for any future flare-ups?

Can you prepare in advance for flare-ups, such as by stocking your freezer with healthy meals you just need to heat up, or ensuring you have a support network you can call on for help?

Flare-ups and negative thoughts

Negative thoughts and emotions during flare-ups are common. When I'm experiencing them it's usual for me to be consumed by the terrible fear that this will become my new normal. These types of negative thoughts and emotions are ones you will likely experience at some point, too – if you haven't already.

Throughout my chronic illness journey there have been times when I have experienced an increase in my baseline symptoms, and I have been forced to adapt and change my life accordingly. So, when I'm flaring up, in pain and exhausted, it can be easy to doubt I'll ever get better. But, to deal with this, I force myself to remember that this flare-up, like all those before it, is temporary. I find it best to take things one step at a time, one day at a time, one hour at a time, one minute at a time, and to remind myself that I have got through this before, and I will again.

It's also essential that I am not masking my negative emotions with forced positivity. The 'Good Vibes Only' type of messaging you will sometimes see around you (usually on social media) is one I strongly disagree with. It is toxic to mask and hide from all negative thoughts, emotions and experiences in order to pretend the positive ones are the only ones present. I truly believe that this strategy is harmful in the long run and can lead to its own mental health issues down the line. We all experience the full spectrum of human emotions, so we should all feel free to be in them, express them, process them and then move on. During a flare-up this is especially important, so we don't waste spoons masking.

Reminder: your flare-ups are temporary. You will return to your baseline once again. Look after yourself by using the management techniques described above and continuing to work hard to prevent the next flare-up (see p. 22), as best you can.

> **Reflections**
>
> What are some thoughts you frequently experience during flare-ups?
>
> Can you find a way to remind yourself that the feelings are likely temporary?

Brain fog

Brain fog is an umbrella term used to describe a range of symptoms that affect your thinking, memory and concentration. Unfortunately, brain frog is incredibly prevalent in the spoonie community because it is linked to several chronic illnesses, conditions and disabilities (such as fibromyalgia, ME/chronic fatigue syndrome, long Covid and lupus, to name just a few), plus it is also a common side effect of many medications, as well as hormonal changes during perimenopause and menopause, for women.

Brain fog can present as the following:

- An inability to focus
- Difficulty finding and/or understanding words
- Struggling with multitasking
- Forgetting things
- Being indecisive
- An inability to follow conversations
- Making simple mistakes
- Feeling confused
- Losing your train of thought
- Slow and/or sluggish thoughts
- Inability to take in and process new information
- Slow recall

If you're experiencing any of these symptoms it's wise to discuss the issue with your doctor to ensure they are aware of it.

Managing brain fog

When it comes to the treatment of brain fog, there are several remedies that you can try at home to improve your situation, in consultation with your doctor. These can include, but are not limited to:

- Getting better-quality sleep (*see* p. 18)
- Reducing stress (*see* p. 21)
- Avoiding alcohol and caffeine
- Doing brain exercises such as puzzles, reading or word and number games
- Managing your chronic illness (*see* p. 17)
- Pacing (*see* p. 63) and rest

Beyond these home remedies, there are other strategies you can try for surviving with brain fog in day-to-day life. These include:

1. Explaining brain fog to those around you
2. Stopping multitasking
3. Making a to-do list
4. Setting alarms

Let's take a look at these in greater depth now.

1. Explain brain fog to those around you

Brain fog is the kind of symptom that can be obvious to those around you. You may trail off in the middle of sentences suddenly, make simple mistakes or forget to do something obvious. For example, if you put the grater in the fridge and the cheese in the dishwasher then others in your household will probably notice something is up.

Even though others will notice something is wrong, they may not understand what is happening. So, having a frank discussion about what brain fog is, what it looks like and what they can do to help you is important. For example, if your brain fog presents as forgetfulness or absent-mindedness it is important for the people you live with to know this. That way you can ask them to double-check things around the home that you may not be confident you have remembered to do, for instance double-checking the stove is turned off or the back door is locked correctly. This is good for everybody's peace of mind.

In fact, if you teach those around you what to look out for with your brain fog then they may begin to notice when something is wrong before you do. That way they'll know to assist you with certain tasks where possible or to remind you of things you need to do, such as taking your medication.

2. Stop multitasking

Splitting your focus is a sure-fire way to make a mistake when you have brain fog. If you try to complete multiple tasks at once it is likely you will forget something or do at least one thing incorrectly. Instead, focus on completing one task at a time correctly before moving on. For some people this is a big adjustment as they are used to juggling lots of things at once. Sometimes it takes practice to focus on one thing at a time, but I have found, from my own experiences and from speaking to other spoonies, that multitasking is virtually impossible with brain fog.

3. Make a to-do list

When living with brain fog, to-do lists are your friend. Keep a running list of things you need to do or create an actual shopping list instead of relying on your memory. List-making is a great way to keep track of all kinds of things, and if you seem to keep misplacing your lists then try getting a planner or diary so they are all in one place, or write them in the notes section of your phone instead.

You can also use a planner or the calendar app on your phone to keep track of all events, medical appointments and social engagements to ensure you are not forgetting anything. This will help you cut down on missed appointments and give you peace of mind.

4. Set alarms

Finally, use alarms on your phone or tablet as reminders. You can set alarms for things like taking your medications, tasks you need to complete that day or events you need to attend. Alarms can be labelled with your own text to remind you what they are for, and you can change the chimes, too. For example, you could use a single ringtone for medication reminders, and another one for event reminders. You can easily set alarms to repeat on certain days, daily, weekly or even multiple times per day.

In my own life I have implemented these brain fog management strategies and found them useful. But it is important that you find systems that work well for you. I suggest you begin by identifying what your brain fog looks like and how it affects you when it occurs (you can use the template symptom tracker in figure 1 on p. 36 to help with this). This will help you highlight any particular problem areas in your daily life, and you can then use the suggestions above to create a plan.

> **Reflections**
>
> How do you experience brain fog?
>
> What's one strategy you can put in place this week to help you cope with brain fog?

Invisible symptoms

A great many of the symptoms related to a chronic illness, condition or disability are invisible, and yet the demands they put on our bodies are very real. That's why living with invisible symptoms is one of the most challenging parts of being a spoonie, and why it is so important to discuss them here.

Invisible symptoms include:

- Pain
- Fatigue
- Brain fog
- Nausea
- Muscle weakness
- Sensory issues

Are invisible symptoms actually invisible?

What's interesting about 'invisible' symptoms – and what people actually living with these invisible symptoms already know – is that many are actually very visible, for anyone who is paying attention, that is. Going back to the list of 'invisible' symptoms above, as a spoonie you may find yourself wondering:

- How can pain be labelled an invisible symptom when I'm wincing and grimacing every five minutes?
- How can fatigue be an invisible symptom when I need to constantly stop and rest?
- How can brain fog be an invisible symptom when I keep trailing off and forgetting what I was saying?
- How can nausea be an invisible symptom when the mere thought of food makes me visibly gag?
- How can numbness and muscle weakness in my legs be an invisible symptom when it makes me stumble while I'm walking?
- How can sensory issues be an invisible symptom when I have to flee the room if it is too loud?

Sometimes I truly believe that these so-called invisible symptoms are named that because people simply don't want to see them.

How to spot invisible symptoms

Visible things a spoonie may do when they have an invisible symptom are:

- Take medications
- Use mobility aids
- Wince or grimace in pain
- Rest often
- Have low energy levels
- Wear support bandages or braces
- Move slowly
- Have slow or slurred speech
- Frequently forget things
- Trail off and be unable to find the right words
- ... and about a thousand other things

Why talking about invisible symptoms is important

Experiencing 'invisible' symptoms can make us spoonies really doubt ourselves. In the past I have thought to myself, multiple times, that if others cannot see my symptoms, maybe I'm not really experiencing them at all. This can lead to us questioning our own reality and lived experiences, which can have dangerous consequences: we may end up avoiding medical care and not correctly managing our own illnesses. This type of self-doubt is truly harmful and should be taken seriously.

It is important for everyone, whether you are a spoonie yourself or not, to understand that a chronic illness, condition or disability doesn't have a specific look; you cannot know what a person is experiencing just by looking at them.

Reminder: hearing comments such as 'But you look so good!' from people around you can be so frustrating, because while we may look 'good' or like we are not ill at all, we are often experiencing symptoms at a level that would put most people in hospital. Often, people will make these types of statements without realising how invalidating they can be. Even though we look good, we do not feel good.

> ## Community column
>
> **What are some frustrating and invalidating things people have said to you?**
>
> '"Wait until you're my age." Sometimes I say, "I'm already in this much pain and I'm only in my 30s, it will only get worse. I'm dreading being your age!"' – Jen
>
> 'I hear, "But there's always something they can do." No, Susan, that's why it's called "chronic".' – Laura
>
> 'Got hit with the "Get well soon" last week and honestly it just gets more infuriating each time.' – KC
>
> '"You're too young." Yes, well, illness doesn't discriminate; that's why we have paediatric hospitals.' – Terri
>
> 'It's the "Have you tried . . . ?" for me.' – Grace

Invisible symptoms are real. Invisible chronic illnesses, conditions and disabilities are real. If you pay attention, you can see them too.

Tracking your symptoms

Tracking your symptoms is a crucial part of living with a chronic illness. Understanding your baseline symptoms will help you manage daily life, while understanding as much as you can about your flare-ups will help you make tweaks to your life to avoid them to some extent.

Keeping a daily log of your symptoms can also provide crucial medical data to your doctors and carers, who can in turn understand more about your body and its needs. Tracking your symptoms can therefore be helpful for anyone with a chronic illness, whether you are new to it or have had one for years.

How do I track my symptoms?

A good way to track your symptoms is to choose daily habits to monitor, as this will help you establish your baseline routine and the symptoms you experience of a daily basis. From here, you will be able to identify when there is a drastic change to your routine, and what may have triggered it.

For example, if you can usually go for a ten-minute walk roughly three times per week, then this is the type of exercise you can do with your baseline symptoms. When you've established this, it'll be easier for you to spot if your symptoms have increased beyond your baseline, i.e. if you're not able to manage the same level of exercise.

To begin, choose which of the daily habits below it makes sense for you to track. Think about what would be helpful for you and your medical team to know (as always, this will vary depending on your individual needs):

- Water intake
- Food intake
- Sleep (duration and quality)
- Pain levels (severity and location)
- Medication taken
- Activity levels
- Exercise log
- Weight changes
- Menstruation
- Blood pressure (using an at-home machine – available at pharmacies or online)
- Mood
- Mental health
- Other symptoms (see table 2 on the next page)

Table 2 Other symptoms you can track

Fatigue	Shivering	Brain fog	Nausea	Cramps	Stiffness	Dry eyes
Joint pain	Swelling	Insomnia	Headaches	Rash	High temperature	Bloating
Migraine	Vision changes	Restless legs	Dizziness	Constipation	Diarrhoea	Heartburn
Vertigo	Balance issues	Numbness	Urine issues	Chest pain	Dry mouth	Sore throat
Acid reflux	Tinnitus	Bruising	Eczema	Hair loss	Light sensitivity	Sweating

To record this data, there are many options. You could use a diary or journal, for example. Any notepad will work, but you may want to check online for a specialised notepad or bullet journal created for spoonies, as these are becoming more and more popular.

Creating your own symptom tracker can be a creative and artistic outlet, too, as you can draw various layouts each week. Or, if that's not really your thing, you can easily print out or buy symptom trackers online. On the following page, there is a template I've created that I use daily to track my symptoms.

Analysing the data

Once you have tracked your symptoms daily for a short while (perhaps a week), it is crucial that you look back on the data and analyse what it is telling you. For example, if you see that you are getting a headache at midday each day and that your water intake is very low by this time, it is safe to suggest that the two may be linked. Once you have noticed this trend or pattern, you can go forward making changes that may help.

In this instance, you can try starting your day with more water and monitor if that helps with the regular headaches. This is a targeted strategy that allows you to make significant progress in managing your own illness without waiting for doctors and medical professionals to tell you what to do and how to do it. This type of pattern recognition

Figure 1 Template symptom tracker

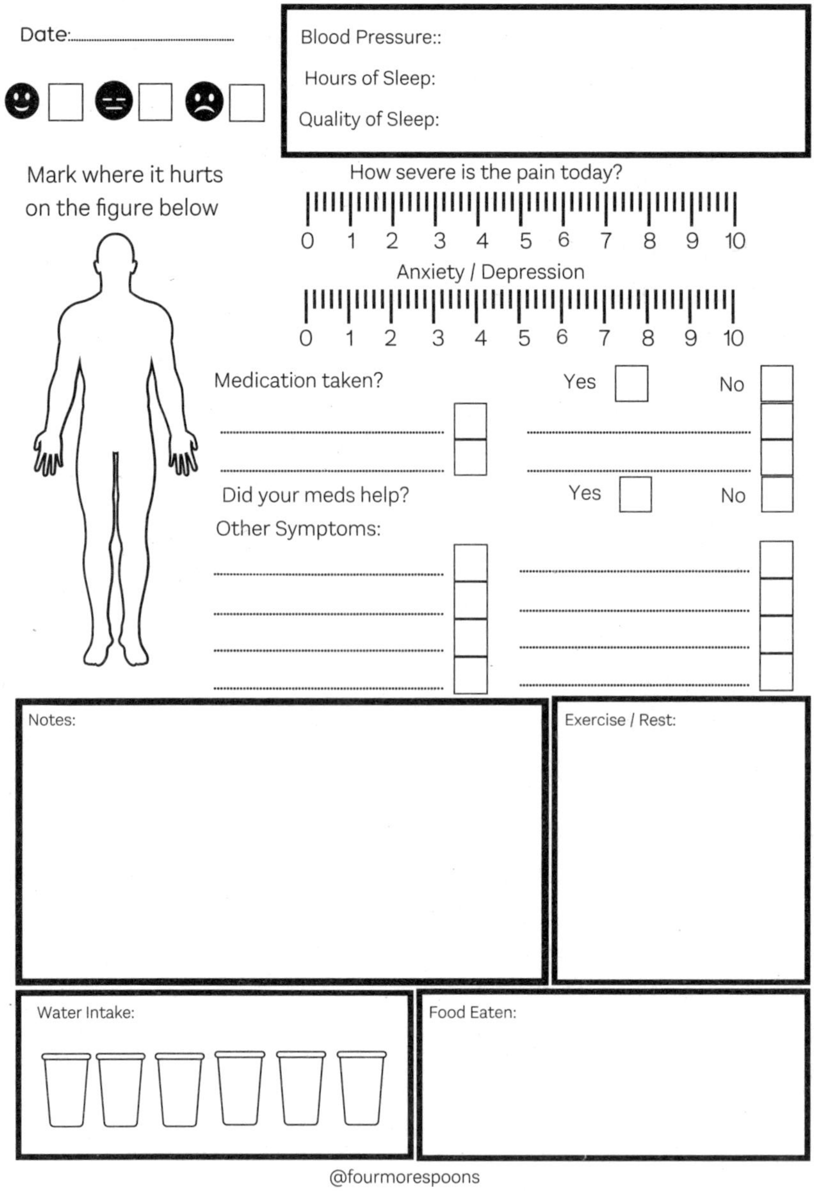

Date:_____

Blood Pressure::
Hours of Sleep:
Quality of Sleep:

Mark where it hurts on the figure below

How severe is the pain today?
0 1 2 3 4 5 6 7 8 9 10

Anxiety / Depression
0 1 2 3 4 5 6 7 8 9 10

Medication taken?   Yes   No

Did your meds help?   Yes   No

Other Symptoms:

Notes:

Exercise / Rest:

Water Intake:

Food Eaten:

@fourmorespoons

is invaluable, especially while waiting for referrals or appointments, as you can save steps when speaking to medical professionals.

By tracking your daily symptoms and other behaviours over a long period of time, you can see if there are any environmental factors that trigger your symptoms, too, or any patterns of behaviour that lead to flare-ups and high-symptom days.

How can tracking your symptoms help with medical appointments?

Continually checking in with yourself through symptom and behaviour tracking is a good way to ensure there are no larger issues that get ignored. If you are having unexplained symptoms that lifestyle changes are not taking care of, this may be a signal that you need to speak with a professional.

With your record to hand, it may be easier to convince your doctor that something is wrong, and you need help. This data collected over time can stop examinations from being delayed and help you get treatment faster. For example, in the scenario with your headaches, above, a doctor may immediately suggest you drink more water, to see if that helps, and then come back in a month. However, because you have already tracked the headaches and your water intake, taken steps to see if that has helped and shown that the headaches are persisting, you can skip forward to a proper examination and treatment options. This speeds up the process and ensures you are not wasting either your or your doctor's time.

Medical gaslighting is where doctors and medical professionals dismiss, downplay or disregard their patients (further details are on p. 89). I have found that providing my doctors with the data I've collected through symptom tracking has forced them to take me and my symptoms more seriously. For the most part, doctors and medical professionals are analytical people; they usually prefer some form of tangible evidence that they can hold in their hands. As there is no real test to distinguish pain levels or fatigue in patients, this type of self-reported data collected over time can be useful to them. It's better to have it and not need it, than to need it and not have it.

Wearable monitors

If paper tracking is not for you, you might consider a wearable device, such as a smart watch, to track certain symptoms. Heart rate and blood pressure monitoring, for example, can be made easier using a wearable device and your doctor may find this data useful for diagnostics. Remember, though, that these types of devices can be wrong, they are not infallible, and your doctor may not be able to use this type of data.

All of the strategies discussed in this chapter require an awareness of what is happening in your body and how it is making you feel. Only then can you try to pre-empt or reduce symptoms, respond appropriately as and when they flare up, and keep a log to help you and your medical care team monitor and analyse what is going on. Doing this should help you to feel slightly more in control of your symptom management and better able to cope with life as a spoonie.

2

Living with pain

Chronic pain is a prominent symptom of many (although not all) chronic illnesses, conditions and disabilities. This chapter will go into the difference between acute and chronic pain, various pain cycles and how to manage chronic pain.

Acute v chronic pain

Pain can usually be broken into two different categories: acute and chronic. Let's look at the difference between the two and how they impact us differently.

Acute pain

Acute pain is pain that begins suddenly – normally as a warning that there is damage or injury to your body that needs to be fixed – and it ends when the source has been treated. The pain of a broken bone is gone once the break has been treated, and therefore this is an example of acute pain.

Aside from broken bones, other causes of acute pain can include, but are not limited to:

- Burns
- Childbirth
- Infection
- Injury

Chronic pain

Chronic pain is defined as pain that lasts beyond the expected recovery period – such as a broken bone that has healed but the pain continues – or pain that is due to a chronic illness, condition or disability. Pain that lasts more than 8 to 12 weeks is often classified as chronic pain. It can affect people in different ways: it can be constant and unending or pain that recurs regularly.

Causes of chronic pain can include, but are not limited to:

- Injuries (but the pain persists past recovery time)
- Illnesses (such as arthritis, cancer or endometriosis)
- Brain chemistry (chemicals in your brain that change the way normal pain signals are sent)
- Ageing
- Genetics (linked to the way we feel pain and the susceptibility of developing chronic pain)

The physical toll that living with chronic pain takes on your body is immense. Unless you experience it yourself, it is unknowable. Before starting my own chronic pain journey, I truly thought I understood what it meant to be in pain. Little did I know!

The pain cycle

When it comes to living with pain, a cycle begins to form. This pain cycle is present for both chronic and acute pain in the body, but it shows up in different ways.

The acute pain cycle

Figure 2 The acute pain cycle

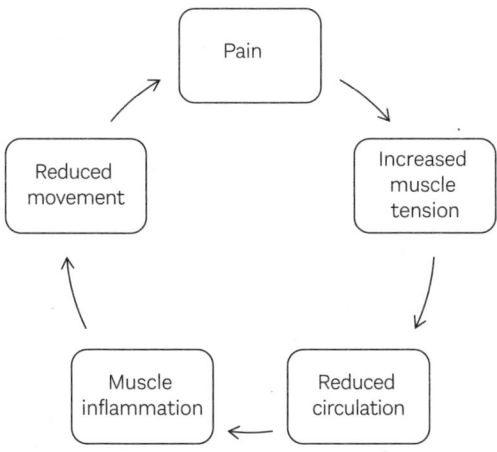

In acute pain patients, different types of intervention can be used to break the acute pain cycle, as shown in figure 2. These include rest, medication, exercise and therapy, such as physiotherapy, medical acupuncture and others. It may take a while to break the cycle, but eventually the pain for acute patients will stop.

The chronic pain cycle

Once pain has persisted beyond the usual recovery period, it moves from acute to chronic and a new cycle for chronic pain begins, as shown in figure 3, on the next page.

At this stage, patients will likely begin to decondition, lose stamina and deal with a certain amount of frustration, fear and stress. All of these issues can compound the chronic physical pain, while the mental health issues also experienced from the cycle can cause changes in your relationships with your loved ones. At all times at least one facet of the chronic pain loop is likely to be impacting the patient and having a huge effect, not only on the body but on the mind and emotions too. Moving in a kind of never-ending loop, the chronic pain cycle can be almost impossible to escape.

Figure 3 The chronic pain cycle

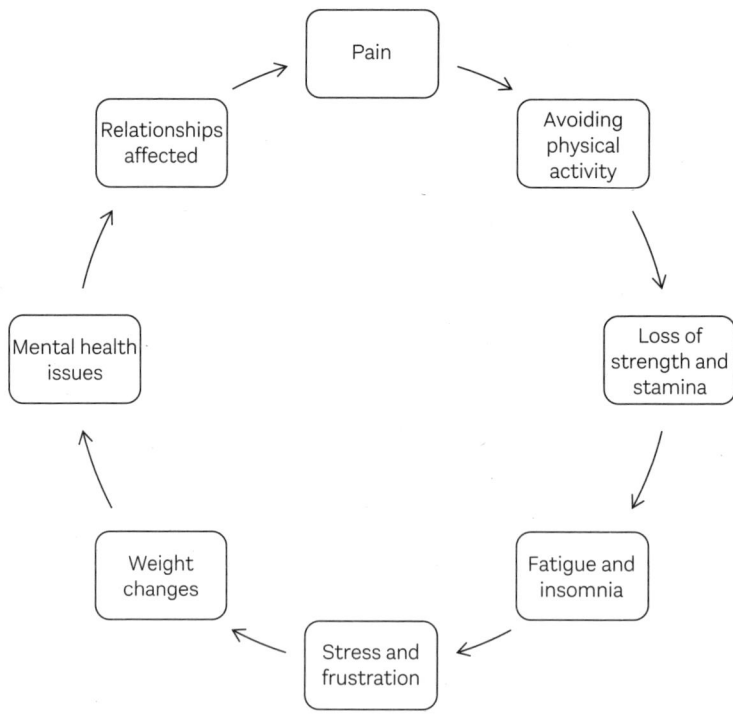

For people with chronic pain, the same interventions used for acute pain can be employed, but they will be less effective. The reasons for this are multiple and varied, but include factors such as genetics, past traumas and many other things we have no control over and that are already baked into us. This is what makes chronic pain so unpredictable.

Unfortunately, it can be very difficult to explain exactly how so many areas of your life can be affected by pain, and what that can feel like. An uncomfortable facet of the chronic pain cycle is how medical professionals perceive it. Often, despite training and education, they cannot comprehend how it can affect you in so many different ways. Unless you are seeing a specialist in pain management, their understanding will likely be reduced to asking you for a number and a description of your pain (see figure 4 on p. 47).

> **Community column**
>
> 'Every single aspect of my life has been affected. That's what people don't get. Until it happens to you, you can have zero concept of it.' – Liv
>
> 'There is so much going on all the time that you can't see. When you ask how we're doing, we say we're "fine" or "just tired" because we couldn't possibly explain every body part that hurts or isn't working quite right, and how immeasurably exhausted we are. It would take too much energy, and you didn't ask for a detailed synopsis, but it's always going on behind the appearance of looking able.' – Ben

The impact of chronic pain

Most people will have an understanding of acute pain, but as we have already examined, the acute pain cycle ends. Chronic pain cycles, on the other hand, continue to wreak havoc on our daily lives. Here is a list of things that chronic pain can take from you:

- Mobility and wellness
- Spontaneity and adventure
- Ambition
- Passion
- Former personality
- Sense of self and identity
- Career/education

It can be easy to allow all of these things to be swept away by chronic pain, but it is so important that you fight that tide. I know: it's just one more thing you need to fight for. But, trust me, it is worth fighting to keep these parts of yourself alive. Your illness and pain is a part of you.

A big part of you. But it is not the only part that matters. Your identity is not your illness, and I want you to remember that.

Managing your illness can be a full-time job but do try to make time for yourself. Take up a new hobby, find something fun to do with friends and family, or try reclaiming something you thought you had lost. The point is that just because chronic pain *can* take those things from you, it doesn't mean that it *has* to take them. You can and should fight to reclaim yourself, even if it is only in some small way.

> ## Community column
>
> 'Before my diagnosis of epilepsy, I was training in martial arts for over 15 years, and I was an avid surfer. Now it's gardening, baking, listening to podcasts and music and spending time with my dog. My zen place!' – Danielle
>
> 'I'm not able to hike like I used to, but photography gets me back outside and appreciating nature!' – Kylie
>
> 'I've always been a crafter and currently it's needle felting because it's something low energy that I can do lying down or sitting, and I really enjoy it.' – Jackie
>
> 'My health has stolen a lot, but I can still have adventures through books.' – Melanie

Reflections

Have you experienced acute pain? Chronic pain? How did they differ from each other?

What has been the biggest impact of chronic pain on your life, and how does it make you feel?

Managing chronic pain

Chronic pain is a complex condition that can and does impact so many areas of your life. Managing it must be done on multiple fronts through various techniques, shown below:

1. Medical management
2. Movement
3. Pacing
4. Sleep
5. Social support

1. Medical management

Managing any and all of your medical conditions is an extremely important step in living with your chronic pain. Whether you believe the two are connected to each other is irrelevant: through better management of your overall health and any other medical issues you may have, you can improve your capacity to cope with your chronic pain.

Something as minor as a common cold or flu can easily exacerbate chronic pain due to the existing inflammation in your body. Overall management of any and all medical conditions, whether chronic or acute, will enable you to better manage your chronic pain.

2. Movement

Exercise and movement are an important step in managing your chronic pain. This can be as simple as a short walk or stretches on the sofa. It can be difficult to do consistently due to pain and other symptoms, but even small amounts of movement can help overall.

Movement may seem like the very last thing you want to do when you are in pain, but in the long run it will help. In the past I have been resistant to this, and it made my pain so much worse. Now I have added gentle stretches into my routine whenever I am able to, and it has made a difference. I do not recommend trying this during a flare-up, however, as it will likely make the pain much worse (ask me how I know...).

3. Pacing

Pacing yourself and resting is and will always be one of the best ways to cope with chronic pain. Attempting to push through and do it all will likely only end in disaster. So, whatever thoughts may be percolating in the back of your mind about needing to do everything, let them go and just slow down. Your body will thank you for it in the end.

4. Sleep

The benefits of good-quality and quantity of sleep cannot be overstated. When your body and mind are not well rested everything bad seems to be compounded and magnified. This is also true of chronic pain. Poor sleep makes your pain feel worse, so use the sleep hygiene tips on p. 18 to help you combat that painsomnia and get a good night's rest.

5. Social support

Ask for help with things you cannot do alone. Whether your support system is your loved ones, carers or even strangers, it is important that you lean on them.

In most cases your loved ones want to help. They hate seeing you in pain and want to make the burden easier, so let them. Carers are there for a reason; it is their job to support and assist you. Charities were set up to help, so use their knowledge and support to lessen the burden on yourself.

The pain scale

Let's talk about the pain scale. This is a numerical scale used in medical settings that is meant to help medical professionals understand the severity of your pain. The patient is asked to give a number, usually between zero and ten, to describe their pain. Many pain scales also use colours or faces to depict the pain level of the patient and can look something like figure 4, below.

Figure 4 The pain scale

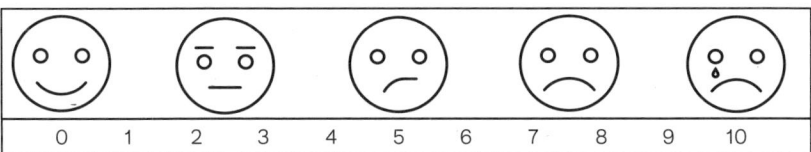

In terms of acute pain, this scale is likely very helpful. Acute pain patients are not 'used to' living with pain and so their reactions will probably look very similar to those shown in the diagram. For example, a ten on the pain scale would probably mean the acute patient is screaming, crying and begging for relief.

However, this type of pain scale is deeply flawed when it comes to chronic pain patients and disabled bodies for two main reasons:

1. People with chronic pain find it hard to verbalise their symptoms and pain level.
2. Pain scales are not designed to support people with chronic pain.

The pain scale was developed as a tool to help people in hospital who are experiencing acute pain (e.g. after surgery) and for children particularly, so it's not overly helpful for those with chronic pain.

Unfortunately, these are systemic rather than individual issues, which can make change difficult to achieve. Let's look at the problems with the current pain scale, and what could be done about them.

1. Use of the numerical scale

Relying on a simple number scale to assess pain is very restricting because it doesn't provide an accurate description of the type of pain the patient is experiencing. By this, I mean people with chronic pain can feel different levels of pain in multiple parts of the body all at once. For example, pain in a person's back may be a four while their head is a nine.

In order to improve upon this design flaw, the scale should ideally be accompanied with descriptive phrases that help the patient draw comparisons to their daily lives. For example, a three might be described as 'patient can continue to do daily tasks with minimal changes' and a six can include the description 'patient requires additional medications to continue to do regular tasks'. This allows for much less subjectivity in describing the level of pain the patient is in and for the medical professional to gain a much better and more nuanced understanding of the situation as a whole.

2. Use of the facial expression diagrams

Medical professionals are trained to look for certain behavioural cues in pain patients in order to accurately assess them. For this reason, the facial expression scale was added to the pain scale.

Unfortunately, a person with chronic pain is unlikely to frown, grimace or cry when they are in a tremendous amount of pain, simply because we are in pain every day. At an optimistic guess, our regular pain will usually start somewhere around a three, and most people living with chronic pain will likely never really be at zero, 'no pain'. This problem is compounded if the patient is neurodivergent and simply doesn't use facial expressions in the ways neurotypical people do and so won't conform to the pictures on the pain scale. They also may have different pain sensitivity and not be able to express the true extent of the problem.

Therefore, despite being in mild, moderate or even severe pain on a daily basis, we spoonies need to continue on with our lives. This means we need to work, cook, clean and care for our families just like everyone else. Unlike everyone else, we do all of these tasks while masking our pain and symptoms as we try to keep going.

I have personally found it incredibly difficult to stop masking my pain, even during medical appointments. Usually this is because it can be difficult to stop and start masking on a whim, and when you get used to masking regularly it can be even harder to stop it, even when you know you need to. Therefore, chronic pain patients can sometimes find themselves in situations where medical professionals simply do not believe we are in the amount of pain we claim to be, and they dismiss us as attention- or drug-seeking. This is incredibly mentally, physically and emotionally damaging and can have long-lasting and far-reaching consequences. (*See* more on medical gaslighting on p. 89.)

In order to rectify this, a complex pain scale should be used in medical settings, especially for chronic pain patients and those who are neurodivergent. This scale would include descriptive language to allow patients to easily identify where they land on the scale (as described on the previous page) and would also include a larger range of facial expressions and numbers continuing past ten. These would allow for a more nuanced view that could help patients and professionals alike.

I believe that education for medical professionals on what chronic pain can look like should be included at all levels of the medical profession, as well as training in understanding the ways chronic pain can affect people's lives. Further training is also needed to understand that not all patients will make faces to express their pain.

Pain descriptions you can use

Pain is different for everybody, but we should be making it as easy as possible to communicate with healthcare professionals who need to understand their patients' symptoms. Table 3 contains some descriptions of the pain you may be experiencing.

Table 3 Terms to describe pain

Sharp	Dull	Burning	Throbbing	Sore
Shooting	Tender	Gnawing	Radiating	Stabbing
Piercing	Cramping	Crushing	Deep	Pulsing
Squeezing	Aching	Searing	Prickling	Itchy

Chronic pain and narcotics

A real hot button issue in the chronic illness community is the use (and misuse) of narcotics in the management of chronic pain. The topic affects so many spoonies, on a global scale, that I believe it is important to touch on this here.

> A brief note on language: opiates specifically refer to narcotics (e.g. oxycodone), while opioids are derived from natural sources, such as poppies (e.g. morphine). Most people use these interchangeably, so for accuracy here I will use the umbrella term 'narcotics'.

First, the World Health Organization found that around 5.8 per cent of the global population used drugs at least once in 2021, around 60 million of which were narcotics. Evidently, research suggests that the use of narcotic medications is a growing concern due to their addictive nature and their long list of severe side effects. Many medical professionals therefore believe they are prescribed too freely and in many countries legislation has been put in place to stop this practice, due to these concerns. This has a far-reaching impact on spoonies who rely on narcotics for pain management, as they may see their necessary medications severely reduced or even cut off.

Second, as narcotics are such a strong medication, the decision to use them or not – if they are offered – is a highly personal one. When prescribed, the person taking narcotics needs to be monitored carefully and reviewed by medical professionals regularly. For some living in chronic pain they are a necessary part of everyday life, while others with long-term pain prefer to avoid them. Many spoonies will need to think about this throughout their chronic pain journey, but there really is no right or wrong answer: it is simply what works best for you.

This section will explore what narcotics are, their use in pain management and the way they are prescribed.

What are narcotics?

Narcotics are a type of powerful painkiller that work by interacting with cells in your brain to relieve pain. Some you may have heard of include:

- Codeine
- Morphine
- Fentanyl
- Oxycodone
- Hydrocodone

In many countries, it is advised that these medications are not prescribed for long-term use, such as in chronic pain patients, or for regular daily use. Any and all patients with a prescription for narcotics are monitored very carefully by their physician and reviewed periodically to ensure there are no long-term issues or negative interactions with other medications being taken by the patient.

When it comes to chronic pain sufferers, narcotics are usually reserved as a measure of last resort, when other medications such as antidepressants, muscle relaxants and anti-inflammatory medications are not working to reduce the amount of pain the patient is experiencing on a regular basis. In this type of scenario, a specialist pain management consultant is likely to be the one to prescribe narcotics, rather than a primary care physician. This is usually due to the complexity of the individual spoonie's medical history and current medical conditions.

When prescribed narcotics, chronic pain patients are normally given the weakest possible drug at the lowest working dosage to ensure the medication is not overly strong. Doctors are likely to slowly adjust the dosage and change medications several times before finding a regimen that works for both doctor and patient. Over time it is likely that a chronic pain patient will try several different medications (both narcotics and other medications) in order to find a combination and dosage that works, but the effectiveness of the medications is likely to change over time.

Are narcotics right for you?

For people living with chronic pain the decision to use or not use narcotics is deeply personal and often difficult to make. It should be based on your individual needs, your circumstances, the advice of your medical team and your own research into the matter. I simply cannot tell you if narcotics are a good idea for you.

For some chronic pain patients, narcotics make the difference between getting out of bed that day or not. These patients will likely decide that taking these strong painkillers is an essential part of their daily life and will continue to take them. In scenarios such as this, patients will need to work closely with their care team, including a pain consultant, primary care physician and prescribing physician, to monitor the effects of such strong medication on their body, their pain and their mental health.

Some people find that narcotics have very little effect on their pain and symptoms, while others find that the negative side effects outweigh the benefits of taking them. These patients may choose to stop taking narcotics altogether or greatly reduce the amount they take. Some people may find that narcotics are best left for high-symptom days and flare-ups, and on days with baseline symptoms only they find that other pain relief methods can get them by.

Common side effects of narcotics

- Constipation
- Nausea
- Vomiting
- Sleepiness
- Confusion
- Dizziness

In high doses or overdose you can suppress the respiratory drive (i.e. you become sleepy/confused, fall unconscious and stop breathing), which can be life-threatening.

Regardless of whether a patient is taking narcotics daily or occasionally, if they have had them for the long term or the short term, it is imperative that all changes to the dosage are closely monitored. Patients must never increase, decrease or abruptly stop taking their medications without consultation with their care team. All changes in medications should be done in small increments, under the direct supervision of medical staff. It is vital to understand that because these medications are so strong, any changes in the dosages that are made too abruptly can have negative and far-reaching side effects. Some medications have potential restrictions on the ability to drive or operate machinery, so please speak to your health provider if you have any concerns.

Personally, I use narcotic painkillers on a daily basis to manage my chronic back pain and fibromyalgia. In my case I tried several different muscle relaxants, anti-inflammatory medications and antidepressants in order to avoid needing these strong painkillers, especially because my pain began at a young age. But despite cycling through dozens of other options, I found very little relief and none that lasted more than a few months at most. Therefore, I made the decision to begin taking narcotic medications in order to live a somewhat normal life.

In my experience I started on very low dose of codeine, then I required a dosage increase until eventually I needed to switch to a more powerful drug. Again, the dosage was carefully adjusted and slowly increased, along with careful monitoring of my overall health and any possible side effects. Over time, between my GP and my pain management team, I have been able to find a combination of several medications (multiple narcotics as well as other medications) that allow me to function.

I would like to emphasise that even with multiple narcotic medications I am never pain free. I live in daily pain despite taking all of the required medications. These strong painkillers barely touch the baseline, surface-level pain I am in, and they come nowhere near touching the pain from a flare-up. However, for me, they are the difference between being able to get out of bed in the morning and not. They are the difference between being able to leave my house and being housebound. For me, narcotics are a necessary evil and despite any side effects I may experience, I will likely always continue to take them.

As with this entire book, this section is written through the lens of my own experience, and I want to make it perfectly clear that I am not encouraging anybody to use narcotics. These medical decisions should be made by consulting your medical care team and not by me. There are very real and very negative side effects to the use of narcotics, including physical effects, mental health issues and the risk of drug addiction.

Community column

'I don't take any narcotics. I've used them in the past and for me the side effects outweigh any relief I might get.' – Louise

'I can see how taking narcotics can be a slippery slope for some, but I've never felt vulnerable to misuse. I think it's vital to recognise that everyone is going to have a different level of tolerance and control. Too many people make narcotics out to be a black-and-white situation but it's not that simple!' – Alli

'I take oxycodone acetaminophen when I rupture an ovarian cyst. The last time this happened it was so bad I was on them for five days. It was awful. I could still feel the pain and it just took the edge off. Coming off them was awful, too. The detox triggered my gastrointestinal disease. But I was beyond grateful to have them. I was grateful to get through the pain.' – L

'I've been taking dihydrocodeine for five years for my pain, [having] tried everything else. I take the same amount daily so that I can get out of bed and go to work. Yes, they can become addictive to some people, but I haven't found that to be true personally.' – Kaz

'I tried tramadol, but it sent me into a totally scary high. I switched to codeine and haven't had any scary side effects. It definitely doesn't take away all the pain, but it makes the chronic pain a bit better.' – Ella

Addiction to narcotics

The issue of narcotic addiction is one of the main reasons the prescription of these powerful medications is so closely controlled via the use of prescription guidelines and government policy. When patients take narcotics long term, their chances of becoming addicted increase greatly. An addiction to narcotics can compound the amount of pain and other symptoms a patient experiences and lead to other profound consequences. This is one of the main reasons doctors are reluctant to prescribe narcotics to people who need them long term, especially as patients will likely get accustomed to their lower doses and require increasingly higher doses over time. Many physicians see even low doses of narcotics as a route to narcotic dependence.

> **Key terms**
>
> Narcotic tolerance: this is the need to take higher and higher dosages of drugs to achieve the same painkiller effect.
>
> Narcotic dependence: this is when you get withdrawal symptoms on reduction of the dose or stoppage of the medication.
>
> Narcotic withdrawal symptoms: these occur only in patients who have developed tolerance.

Signs of narcotic addiction include:

- Craving narcotics and thinking constantly about your next dose
- Taking more than the prescribed dosage, even though you are getting bad side effects
- Taking narcotics to 'feel calm' or 'help get to sleep', or any other reason than pain relief
- Experiencing withdrawal effects when you stop taking them
- Engaging in risky behaviour to get more drugs

It is worth noting that this list of the signs of narcotic addiction is not a complete one. There may be others, and if you believe yourself or someone you know is experiencing an addiction you should seek help immediately. Speak to a pharmacist, nurse or doctor about how to safely stop taking narcotics and remove unused medications from the home.

Reminder: It is extremely dangerous to attempt to abruptly stop taking narcotics. Dosage reduction should be done slowly and under the supervision of medical professionals. Quitting by 'going cold turkey' can cause harm.

Signs of narcotics withdrawal

1. Shivers
2. Trouble sleeping
3. Increased pain
4. Nausea
5. Vomiting
6. Sweating
7. Diarrhoea
8. Aching body
9. Irritability
10. Mood swings

Reflections

Can you use some of the terms in table 3 (page 49) to describe your pain more accurately?

What are your views on narcotics use to manage chronic pain?

3
Living with fatigue

Fatigue is a type of extreme exhaustion. It's a feeling of tiredness that simply cannot be remedied with rest and sleep, a bone-deep weariness that saps your energy and any motivation you have to be productive. Fatigue can make it difficult to move, to think and to do basic tasks like eat and drink.

Unfortunately, fatigue is linked to several chronic illnesses, conditions and disabilities, so it's a fairly common symptom in the spoonie community. Let's explore it further.

Causes of fatigue

In order to successfully manage your fatigue, you and your doctor must first identify where it stems from so that you can begin to make tweaks accordingly. Research has found that the causes of fatigue usually fit into one of three main categories:

1. Lifestyle factors – our habits and behaviours
2. Physical health conditions – due to genetics or our lifestyle/environmental factors
3. Mental health conditions – due to genetics, physical health conditions, substance issues or past history

Table 4 shows common factors that can lead to fatigue, but please note that is not a complete list.

Table 4 Common factors that can lead to fatigue

Lifestyle factors	Physical health factors	Mental health factors
Physical exertion	Anaemia	Anxiety
Lack of decent-quality sleep	Arthritis	Depression
Weight issues	Fibromyalgia	Seasonal affective disorder (SAD)
Substance use	Chronic fatigue syndrome/ME	Bipolar disorder
Caffeine usage	Under-/overactive thyroid	Post-traumatic stress disorder (PTSD)
Poor nutrition	Insomnia	Schizophrenia
Stress	Eating disorders	
	Autoimmune disorders	
	Congestive heart failure	
	Cancer	
	Diabetes	
	Kidney/liver disease	
	Chronic obstructive pulmonary disease (COPD)	
	Emphysema	

Any of the factors listed above can cause fatigue in anybody, but when multiple factors occur in one person it can be difficult to pinpoint, and therefore treat, the exact cause. This is why it is so important that you speak with your medical care team if you are experiencing fatigue alongside your other symptoms, so they can more precisely identify the possible causes and therefore understand the treatment you need.

To help identify the cause/s of your fatigue your doctor will need to ask you several questions to find out more about:

- Your fatigue itself: when it started; if it ever gets better or worse; how it affects your daily life.

- Other symptoms you may experience: be honest here and list every symptom that you do experience (even if you feel it's minor or irrelevant to fatigue), because all your symptoms combined could point to a particular illness or disorder.
- Other medical conditions you may have: it is essential that your doctor understands whether your fatigue is an expected symptom of another illness or an unexpected symptom from an undiagnosed condition.
- Your lifestyle and stressors: your doctor will need information about your sleep, activity, eating and drinking habits in order to determine whether or not there may be a lifestyle change you could make to help lessen the fatigue.
- Medications you're taking: your doctor will need to know if fatigue is an expected side effect of any medication you are currently taking and determine whether this medication needs to be changed completely or tweaked to reduce the side effects you are experiencing.

After gaining as much information from you as they can, your doctor may need to carry out further testing to see if there are any medical or mental health conditions causing your fatigue (which can then be managed better to eliminate the fatigue). If none are found, then the suggested causes of fatigue are thought to be lifestyle factors, so many doctors will prescribe lifestyle changes – such as better-quality sleep, weight loss and exercise – as a default prescription.

Managing fatigue

Regardless of the cause of your fatigue there are some universal fatigue management techniques that you can try. We can call these strategies 'the four Ps of fatigue management'. They are:

1. Problem-solving
2. Planning
3. Prioritising
4. Pacing

1. Problem-solving

A straightforward way to manage your fatigue is by identifying any stressors and triggers that may be adding to your overall levels of fatigue and thinking of some ways to reduce or eliminate them. For example, if my weekly grocery shopping trip is adding to my fatigue and causing me to spend spoons I really do not have to spare, I would need to think of ways I can solve this problem. The easiest solution would be to switch to online grocery shopping or get someone else to help me with this task. While it may seem obvious, it is imperative that you can identify areas of your life that are adding to your fatigue and solve the problem in new and often creative ways.

2. Planning

Planning ahead by knowing what you want to achieve during your day or week can help you manage your overall levels of fatigue. This can include organising your time so that instead of attempting and failing to carry out large tasks all at once, you break them down into smaller and more manageable chunks and tackle each one individually. This will take some forward planning to ensure you achieve everything you wish to, but it can be done with some effort and perseverance on your part. In our grocery shopping example, planning ahead to ensure you have someone available to help would be a good idea.

3. Prioritising

It is critical to prioritise your to-do list. Important tasks should be made a priority so you don't end up doing too much all at once. To help you prioritise, ask yourself the following:

- Does this need to be completed today?
- Is it really necessary for me to do this?
- Can someone else do this for me?
- Can I get help with certain aspects of this task?

Let's say your to-do list has three items on it: your hospital appointment, grocery shopping and buying some new shoes. If you organise this list by priority then it becomes obvious your appointment is unavoidable and essential; this is where you should spend your spoons. Your grocery shopping can be delegated to someone else (either a loved one, carer or delivery service) and shoe shopping is your lowest-priority item. This can be done at another time (if possible) or exclusively online (if it is urgently needed). Modifying your to-do list using prioritisation is a good way to ensure you are not doing too much and compounding your fatigue.

4. Pacing

Pacing is all about ensuring you are not using all of your limited spoons in one go but spreading them out as much as possible to complete your prioritised tasks. Finding time to rest and replenish your spoons is an essential part of living with and managing fatigue. Check out the next chapter for more information regarding pacing, what it is and how it can help in your daily life.

> **Reflections**
>
> Have you and your medical team pinpointed the cause of your fatigue?
>
> How could you implement the four Ps of fatigue management into your daily life?

4

The art of pacing yourself

What is pacing?

Pacing is a strategy that allows individuals to balance time spent on activity and resting to boost functionality.

Living with a myriad of physical symptoms can be tough. It is a balancing act trying to conserve energy and continue living a somewhat normal existence. In order to do this, pacing yourself is a necessary part of daily life (see p. 170 in the Lifestyle section for more). How you do this will likely look very different for us all, as it's dependent on factors such as your job, your family and your home life.

I want to acknowledge right from the start two key things about pacing. First, pacing is a privilege. Second, pacing and resting do not make you lazy. Let me explain . . .

1. Pacing is a privilege

Conserving your energy through rest is a privilege. Being able to live a life where you do not need to work – or where you can prioritise pacing over your career – is a luxury that many disabled and chronically ill people simply do not have. Many are also not able to prioritise their energy over other obligations, such as raising a family, and so many spoonies are forced to push past their own limits and inevitably do too much.

My best advice is that wherever it is possible to pace yourself and conserve energy, then please do; it will really help you in the long run.

2. Pacing and resting do not make you lazy

Additionally, let's be clear: resting does not make you lazy! Instead, resting and pacing are necessary to keep you going for longer. Spoonies require more rest than the average, able-bodied person. Full stop. I won't be taking any arguments about this.

So, now we have these two key points out of the way, let's discuss how to rest and pace successfully.

How to successfully rest and pace

This section will look into some of the pacing and resting strategies that can help you manage your chronic illness, condition or disability. In an ideal world you would be able to implement all of these steps into your life immediately, but any progress, however small, is better than nothing. To support pacing you can:

1. Schedule rest
2. Prioritise your to-do list
3. Set boundaries
4. Listen to your body
5. Switch off

1. Schedule rest

It may seem strange to schedule a rest day in your calendar, but if that is literally what you need to do, open your calendar now and add it in. It is very common to have such a busy schedule with work and other obligations that you may feel you simply do not have the time to rest.

However, scheduling a day off in your calendar will force you to keep some time free of other people's requests and other commitments and carve out some space for yourself.

By scheduling rest days throughout your week and month you can ensure you are setting aside enough time to recharge your batteries regularly. Even if you cannot find an entire day to rest, set aside a few hours.

Also take a look at what events, appointments or activities are scheduled in your calendar, and make sure you are taking the appropriate amount of time before and after these to rest. It is essential to rest before events, and depending on how tiring the actual event is, you may need to take a few hours or days to recover afterwards, too. Taking the initiative to plan this ahead of time can make the event more enjoyable, as you'll have enough spoons in hand to enjoy it, and it means that you can hopefully avoid overscheduling yourself and burning out.

2. Prioritise your to-do list

It's vital that you get good at learning what your needs are and then prioritising them. This is a message I'll repeat throughout the book, for good reason.

Understanding your needs comes from self-reflection and introspection, as everybody's priorities are different. For the most part, though, you probably know what it is you value in your life and what you want to do more or less of. When you've identified which events and activities are the most important to you and your family, do those first. Then spend time resting and see if you can do the less-essential ones afterwards.

Begin with what is the most pressing or important to you so that, if you need to stop, you are in a position to do so without skipping these key tasks. Save your spoons on high-symptom days by putting off non-essential tasks, and on low-symptom days carry out any remaining tasks while at the same time being careful not to push yourself too far and overdo it.

Knowing and learning your priorities can be difficult: it takes a certain amount of self-reflection, but it is an important part of being able to pace yourself carefully, making it time well spent in the long run.

3. Set boundaries

Be very clear to those around you about your boundaries. When it comes to declining invitations this can be difficult, because even if we want to attend certain activities and events, sometimes our bodies simply will not let us. So, in order to combat any guilt about this, be clear with those around you and explain why you may not be able to attend their events. Once you have set these boundaries and said no to an event, make sure you do not back down from your position. It is your right to say no to things because you need to.

4. Listen to your body

On a similar point, it is so important that you listen to what your body is telling you it needs. Pain and high symptoms can be your body's way of telling you to rest. You know yourself best, so tune in and act accordingly. When you are doing too much, pushing yourself past your natural limitations, it will become clear very quickly.

Sometimes listening to your body can mean cancelling plans at the last minute, leaving an event early or missing out on something you really would like to do. Unfortunately, this is the unfair reality of living with a chronic illness, condition or disability. Learn your limits and try not to push them too far, too often, if it can be avoided.

5. Switch off

When resting, it can be highly beneficial to switch off and unplug from screens and constant input. While vegging out on the sofa or scrolling endlessly can seem like a great way to rest, sometimes a peaceful and tranquil hour or two without screens can do wonders, too. Find the right balance for you and experiment with periods of digital detoxing.

It's also worth noting that just because you are sitting still, that does not mean you are resting. You can sit on the sofa but continue to worry about everything you need to do, get caught up in making a mental to-do list or fret over the fact that you are not being productive. This isn't really resting. Resting doesn't just mean sitting still: it can be anything that takes your mind off your worries and allows you to relax.

Reminder: high-quality rest can be anything you want it to be, so long as you are taking time for yourself, recharging your batteries and enjoying yourself.

Community column

'Ideally I think it's best to be present in the moment of rest and not think about work or whatever else . . . but the thing is it's so hard to do because I feel like society has programmed us to be go go go all the time.' – Flo

'I like to rest by watching TV on the couch, preferably with a blanket and a cat.' – Heather

'My mother-in-law asked me, "what do you do when you are resting?" For me, resting is doing nothing.' – Marguerite

'I prefer to rest through travel.' – Kristin

'For me, resting is my bed, Netflix, pain meds, chocolate and a can of juice. And no children!' – Watson

Reflections

Are you getting enough rest?

What could you be doing differently to ensure you are pacing yourself?

Should I rest or participate today?

Learning what pacing is and understanding how to achieve high-quality rest is great. But at the same time you need to have tools to help you identify when it is time to rest and when it is OK to participate. In this section I'll be sharing two self-assessment tools that I use to help me determine when I need to rest and when I can join in with activities.

Tool one: self-assessment for resting

I have created a three-step strategy that I use on a daily basis to assess myself and decide if today will be a rest day or not. This is a fairly simple (and probably quite obvious) checklist strategy, but it is helpful to have it spelled out like this, in a way you can refer to easily when in doubt. Sometimes, a back-to-basics approach is the best way to relearn behaviour and force it to become second nature.

So here's my three-step strategy for deciding: should I rest today?

1. Self-assessment
2. Check your calendar
3. Prioritise

1. Self-assessment

The first step is to make an accurate and honest self-assessment of yourself. I have formulated four easy questions that I ask myself to help me decide if I should rest:

  I. How am I feeling right now?
  This is the very first question to answer. It may be as simple as saying 'good' or 'bad', or a more detailed answer, but generally speaking knowing how you are feeling at the moment is a good place to start. Personally, if I am not feeling so great at the current moment, I know adding an activity or outing on top of that will only cause me to feel worse, either physically or mentally, and

so I decide not to participate. Once I have answered this initial, and very important, question, I move on to the rest of the self-assessment.

II. Do I have the physical energy to do [insert relevant activity]?
Answer either 'yes' or 'no'.

III. Do I have the mental energy to do [insert relevant activity]?
Answer either 'yes' or 'no'.

IV. If I do [insert relevant activity] will I cause myself a flare-up/increase my symptoms?
Answer either 'yes' or 'no'.

A simple 'yes' or 'no' answer to these questions is often all I need to know when deciding if I want to participate. For example, if the answer is 'no', I do not have the physical or mental energy today, I would not participate. However, if I feel OK and have the spoons to carry out tasks, and I don't think they will cause a flare-up, I can move on to the next step of the process.

2. Check your calendar

The next stage is to check your calendar. This can help you decide if today will be a rest day or not. For example, if today is Sunday and I have a day out planned for Tuesday that will involve using lots of energy, I will need to carefully consider the next few days. As there is a buffer day in between, I can carry out small, easy-to-do tasks on Sunday and leave Monday as a rest day ready for Tuesday. This would mean I need to ensure that I do not push myself too far on Sunday and make any final preparations as early as possible to ensure Monday is a low-activity, low-stress and restful day.

3. Prioritise

The final step of this strategy is a familiar one: prioritise! (See, I told you I'd keep mentioning it a lot.)

Often my ability to rest is decided based upon the urgency of the tasks I need to carry out. If I am unable to put off or postpone certain tasks or appointments (usually medical appointments and procedures) then I will get as much rest as possible beforehand, as well as after, while asking others around me for help wherever possible; for example, with errands like grocery shopping or cleaning tasks. Chores inside the house that need doing will take a back seat to a medical appointment outside the home, because one is a clear priority in terms of spending my limited number of spoons.

My best advice is to only attempt to do half of the tasks that you think you can do on any day, and when you reach the halfway point or any other natural stopping points, stop, rest and assess your available spoons. Ask yourself if it is safe to continue working (will you be using too many spoons if you continue and/or will it cause a flare-up?) or do you need to rest?

It is vitally important that you are honest with yourself and never try to push past your body's natural limitations. You're the one feeling the consequences of these actions, nobody else. You need to pause and reassess yourself and your needs at every available opportunity.

Tool two: self-assessment for participating

When living with chronic pain or other physical symptoms, it can be difficult to decide whether or not participating in a certain event or activity is the best option for you. It can be difficult, for example, to know if going bowling for your friend's birthday is a good idea or not.

However, I've created a second simple self-assessment tool – see figure 5 on the next page – to help visualise my needs and determine what activities are a good option for me or not.*

---

* In my own experience, pain is the main symptom that determines whether I can participate in certain activities. But if pain is not your main concern or symptom (for example, you might be more affected by fatigue or muscle weakness), you can adjust the questions in the diagram to better reflect your own needs.

I personally like to make this self-assessment at least a couple of days before the event and once more on the day of the event, but you should feel free to adapt this tool to your own needs.

Additionally, while it may be difficult to know how long your recovery time will take, sometimes we can get a good idea by looking at how strenuous an event or activity it is, and by understanding your usual recovery time. For example, if I spend the day walking around the zoo I will probably take days to recover, whereas if I spend an hour walking around a shopping centre I will probably only take a few hours to recover.

Be honest about your current condition and how long your recovery usually takes in terms of pain and other symptoms, then make your decision on that basis, even if it means missing out on things you want to do.

Figure 5 Self-assessment

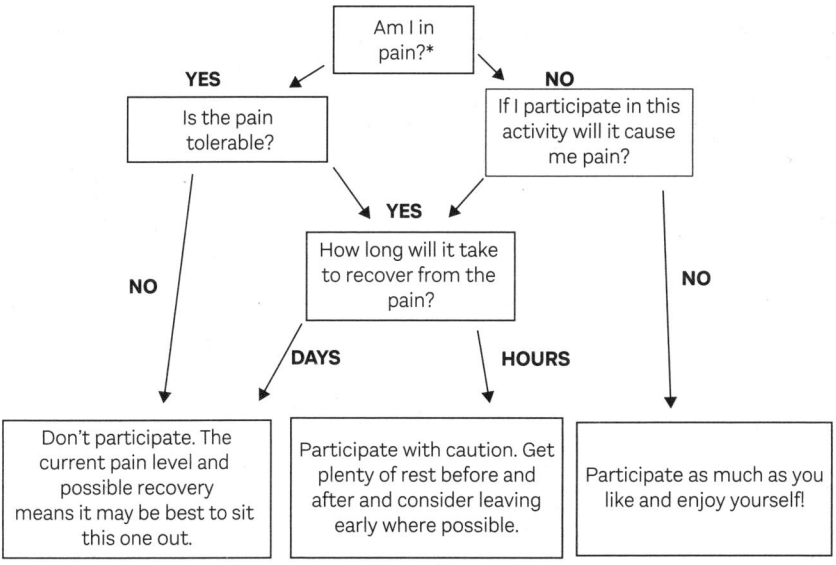

* Switch out pain with any symptom of your choice to adjust this diagram to your own needs.

The boom–bust cycle

The boom–bust cycle (also known as the push–crash cycle) is where a low-symptom or 'good' day occurs and as a result you end up overdoing it, pushing yourself too hard and too fast and having a flare-up. You are forced to rest and recover and eventually this will lead to another low-symptom day, and so on. Unfortunately, many people, me included, do not learn from the experience, and end up repeating the cycle again (and again, and again...).

Figure 6 Boom-bust cycle

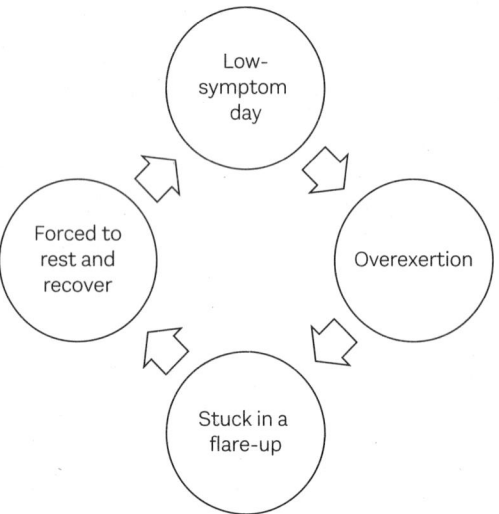

It can be especially difficult to break this cycle if your good days are very rare, because it can feel like you need to take full advantage of the few good days you get, even though this results in a flare-up. Often, people do not realise that they are even in the cycle, and this makes it all the more difficult to escape it, meaning people can be unwittingly stuck in it for years.

> **Community column**
>
> 'It took me three years to break this [boom–bust] cycle. Lots of things helped but mainly it was finally accepting my limits and that I was genuinely unwell and none of this was normal.' – Charlotte

I have found the best way to break this boom–bust cycle is by employing all of my pacing tactics of conserving spoons, even on good days (see p. 65). By pacing myself, saving energy where possible and spreading out tasks over several days instead of a few hours, I can avoid overexertion and the resultant flare-up.

Reflections

Have you ever been stuck in a boom–bust cycle?

What can you be doing differently to ensure you are not stuck in this type of cycle?

2

Mental health

1. Depression and anxiety   77
2. Medical gaslighting   89
3. Distancing yourself from unsupportive people   103
4. Imposter syndrome and self-doubt   115
5. Burnout   121

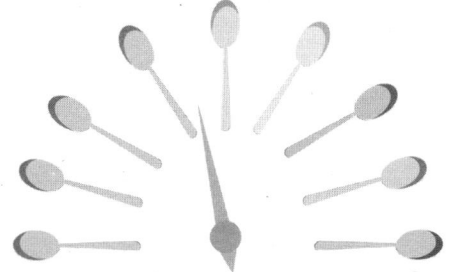

1
Depression and anxiety

Living with a chronic illness, condition or disability means that mental health problems are much more likely. This is because being a spoonie brings higher-than-average risks of isolation, stress and even discrimination, all of which can lead to mental health issues.

Mental health problems in turn can unfortunately seriously affect your ability to manage your chronic illness, condition or disability, so you can at times become stuck in a cycle of physical health and mental health issues. This can cause symptoms throughout your body, and it can be hard to tell which came first.

This chapter will therefore explore the link between chronic illness and mental health – looking specifically at depression and anxiety, as this relationship is proven to be closely linked.

Reminder: there is no shame in having mental health issues and you can and should seek professional advice and counselling wherever possible.

Depression

Depression is so much more than just the feelings of sadness that can happen to anyone throughout their daily lives. It is more of a persistent low mood that can last weeks or months (or longer), rather than just a few days. Many people still dismiss depression as a trivial issue, something that's easy to overcome and move on from, but in actuality it is a very real and serious health condition.

When it comes to living with depression, alongside your chronic health conditions, the symptoms of your depression, such as listlessness, poor sleep and changes in appetite, can exacerbate your already existing physical symptoms.

You see, when living with a chronic illness, our bodies are finely tuned ecosystems that require constant maintenance and upkeep. A change in mood can cause a change in behaviour, which can lead to a change in our bodies. It is therefore not difficult to understand that the mind and the body are interconnected, and that changes in one will affect the other.

Feelings of listlessness, for example, can lead to poor management of your chronic illness, condition or disability. For example, perhaps you'll skip the physical activity you need to do to keep flare-ups at bay. At the other end of the spectrum, thoughts of self-harm or suicide from your depression can be particularly dangerous if you have access to strong medications and painkillers for the management of your chronic pain. That is why it is so important for spoonies to take care of our mental health as well as our physical health.

Symptoms of depression

Identifying the symptoms of depression and understanding that they go beyond 'just sadness' is essential. Knowing what to look out for in yourself and your loved ones may mean that diagnosis and treatment happen as soon as possible. This can be the difference between life and death.

Symptoms of depression can include:

- Feelings of sadness
- Feelings of hopelessness
- Feelings of anger or irritability
- Brain fog symptoms
- Changes in appetite (eating too much or not enough)
- Changes in sleep patterns (too much or too little)
- Low energy
- Low mood
- Thoughts of self-harm or suicide
- Feeling worthless/low self-esteem
- Losing interest in activities you once enjoyed
- Low sex drive
- Physical aches and pains

If you are experiencing symptoms of depression for extended periods of time it is essential that you speak with your medical care team in order to get help. Your doctor will ask you how you are feeling and try to discern any potential causes for your depression. It can be extremely difficult to open up and talk frankly about your situation, but it is important for both your mental and physical health that you do so as best as you can.

Reminder: opening up about your health is the only way you can get the diagnosis you need and receive the correct treatment.

Different types of depression

It is also important to note that there are many different types of depression with varying underlying causes and effects on your body. Let's run through some of the types of depression and what they are.

Clinical depression

This term simply means a doctor has given you a diagnosis of depression.

Depressive episode

A formal name for depression when doctors make a diagnosis. These can be labelled mild, moderate or severe.

Recurrent depressive disorder

Once you have had at least two depressive episodes, the doctor may say you have recurrent depressive disorder. This essentially means your depressive episodes can and do happen repeatedly. This can also be labelled mild, moderate or severe.

Reactive depression

If your depression seems to be triggered by difficult life events it can be labelled as reactive. This means the depression is a response to some sort of stimulus, most commonly life events. These could include money stress, divorce or a death in the family, as well as many other things.

Dysthymia

This is where you are experiencing mild depression over two years. It is also known as chronic depression or persistent depressive disorder. The emphasis here is that the depression is mild but long-lasting.

Cyclothymia

This is where you experience persistent unstable moods with extreme highs and lows, but these periods are not long enough or severe enough to qualify for a bipolar diagnosis.

Bipolar disorder

Formerly known as manic depression, bipolar disorder involves cycling between periods of mania and depression. Mania typically consists of lots of energy, lack of sleep, poor decision-making, risky behaviour (such as gambling, drinking and taking recreational drugs) and sometimes psychosis. These phases of mania and depression take place over weeks and months rather than days and hours.

Psychotic depression

This is where you are experiencing delusions or hallucinations alongside your depressive episode. A hallucination means you may see, hear, smell, taste or feel things that are not real. This is different from a delusion, which means that you might believe things that are not matching reality.

Pre- or postnatal depression

Prenatal depression is experienced during pregnancy, also known as antenatal depression. Postnatal depression occurs after becoming a parent and can affect any gender.

Seasonal affective disorder (SAD)

This is a type of depression experienced during certain seasons of the year, due to the weather conditions. Energy and mood may dip when it gets colder or warmer and you may experience changes in eating and sleeping patterns too. This will occur at the same time every year and is most common in the winter months.

Treatment options for depression

Treatment for depression can involve a combination of several different things at once, usually depending on the type of depression you have and how severe it is. Most common are lifestyle changes, talking therapy and medications.

- Lifestyle changes can include anything from increased exercise and better nutrition to meditation to help treat your depression.
- Cognitive behavioural therapy (CBT) is a talking therapy used to treat depression. It can be done in person, online or over the phone. It is usually prescribed for mild depression.
- Antidepressants are usually employed for more severe types of depression and may also be used in combination with other remedies.

> **Reflections**
>
> Have you ever experienced symptoms of depression?
>
> If so, how have they affected your physical health?

Anxiety

Anxiety symptoms can also be a common part of life with a chronic illness, condition or disability. Fears about the future, finances (see Part Three, p. 133), treatment options and accessibility are all common concerns for spoonies, and negative thought patterns surrounding these can lead to anxiety symptoms. These may include feelings of worry, unease or dread and can be labelled mild, moderate or severe.

Anxiety coupled with physical health conditions and disabilities can be difficult to live with, as they can feed into each other and make both worse, in exactly the same way that symptoms of depression can exacerbate symptoms from chronic illnesses, as discussed on p. 78.

Different types of anxiety

Let's begin by discussing some of the most common types of anxiety and the symptoms that are commonly associated with them.

Generalised anxiety disorder (GAD)

Generalised anxiety disorder can be described as feelings of unease, fear and worry, usually in certain, specific situations. GAD is a chronic, long-term condition that is not triggered by a single event but by a wide range of different events and situations throughout the person's life. For example, it is expected that someone would have some feelings of anxiety at an important job interview or before receiving significant medical test results. At times like these it is normal and even expected that you feel some kind of anxiety-related symptoms.

Most of the time, people with GAD will experience anxiety symptoms during stressful situations but also in everyday ones. For example, as well as experiencing anxiety waiting for medical test results they would feel anxious making a simple phone call or going shopping. For these people, anxiety-inducing situations are usually everyday stresses and as soon as an anxious thought is resolved another one is ready to take its place.

It is unclear what the exact cause of generalised anxiety disorder is but there are several factors that can contribute to having it:

- Genetics
- Personal history (domestic violence, child abuse, bullying, etc.)
- Long-term health conditions
- Substance abuse

It is also important to note that you can have anxiety for no apparent reason at all.

Treatment options for generalised anxiety disorder

There are several treatment options for generalised anxiety disorder that can help. Often they are used in combination with each other:

- Talking therapies such as cognitive behavioural therapy are usually the first step in treating anxiety. Discussing the issue and learning techniques to reshape your thoughts can be effective for all types of anxiety.
- Medication can also be helpful for those with GAD. These may include selective serotonin reuptake inhibitors (SSRIs), beta blockers or benzodiazepines. SSRIs are used to treat a variety of disorders including depression, anxiety, post-traumatic stress disorder (PTSD) and obsessive compulsive disorder (OCD). Beta blockers may be useful for short-term use and benzodiazepines are normally prescribed sparingly due to the risk of addiction.

Social anxiety

This is a type of anxiety surrounding social situations and is a long-term phobia that manifests as anxiety. This is commonly seen as early as the teenage years and can continue throughout the person's life. Some spoonies experience this type of anxiety due to the fact they may require additional support in social settings, making them fear they are in the spotlight more than their peers.

Many who suffer from social anxiety find it very distressing to be put into social situations, and this can manifest as extreme shyness and a lack of self-esteem and self-confidence. Symptoms of social anxiety can include:

- Worry regarding things like meeting new people, having conversations or speaking on the phone
- Avoiding social settings like eating out, going to pubs, or group activities
- Constantly stressing that you have done something embarrassing
- Blushing, sweating or stuttering when talking in social situations
- Feeling judged or watched when others look at you while doing something
- Avoiding eye contact
- Fear of being criticised or called out in some way
- Sweating
- Trembling
- Heart palpitations
- Panic attacks

It is fairly common for someone with social anxiety to also have generalised anxiety disorder and other mental health issues. Neurodivergent people also commonly experience social anxiety as part of their disability.

Treatment options for social anxiety

Ways to help with your social anxiety can include things like:

- Attempting to understand more about where your anxiety stems from, so you could try writing down your thoughts and behaviours in social situations.
- Breathing exercises and meditation can help calm your mind and body and reduce your overall stress.
- Breaking down tasks into smaller and more manageable chunks can help you to follow through on social situations. For example, you can break down the steps of getting ready to go out into: take a shower, do your hair, pick an outfit. By focusing on each individual task, the thought of going out becomes more manageable.
- Therapies such as CBT are also recommended for social anxiety.
- Medications like SSRIs may also be prescribed for social anxiety.

Health anxiety

Health anxiety is where a person spends all of their time worrying about their health; they worry they are ill or will become ill and these thoughts begin to take over their life. Spoonies with chronic health conditions spend more time than most people worrying about their health and this can easily become obsessive and morph into health anxiety.

Some symptoms of health anxiety include:

- Constantly worrying about your health
- Frequently checking for lumps, bumps or bruises (and any other physical signs of illness)
- Seeking constant reassurance that you are not ill
- Fear that medical professionals have missed something
- Obsessing over health information, medical diagnoses or various conditions online

- Avoiding things to do with illnesses, like medical dramas or watching certain news segments
- Acting as though you are ill when you are not, such as avoiding physical activity or constantly monitoring health stats

Having any type of anxiety can cause physical symptoms like headaches, dizziness or heart palpitations, and people with health anxiety may take this as proof they are truly ill and continue to obsess over their health, creating a cycle, as shown in figure 7, below.

Figure 7 Health anxiety cycle

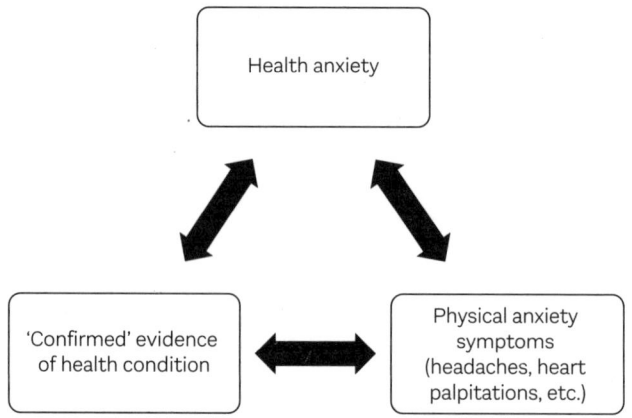

Treatment options for health anxiety

Keep a diary and track how often you check your body for signs of illness, look up health information or seek reassurance from those around you. Once you know this baseline of information, set a goal of gradually reducing these types of behaviours each week. Keep these changes in gradual increments, as stopping suddenly can lead to relapses and further anxiety. For example, if you find yourself checking your pulse and blood pressure three times per day, slowly reduce it to twice per day and then gradually down to only a couple of times per week.

Challenge the anxious thoughts when you have them. In your diary, write down the anxious thoughts you commonly have about your health and then think of more balanced and reasonable thoughts to counter these points. If you are struggling to think of the balanced side of the argument, ask for help countering each one from a friend or family member. Using someone you trust can help you break the cycle of anxious thoughts by introducing more rational ones. For instance, if you constantly find yourself worrying that a headache is a brain tumour, look up and write down other causes for headaches, such as excessive screen time and dehydration. Consider whether any of these factors could be the cause of your headache rather than jumping to the worst possible conclusion.

Keeping busy is also so important for health anxiety. Distracting yourself when anxious thoughts come up can be a good way to avoid giving in to anxious behaviours. For example, if you find you want to constantly check your blood pressure and heart rate, try distracting yourself by calling a friend, going for a walk or even trying a new hobby.

Once you feel ready, it is important that you begin to gradually introduce the things you have been avoiding. For example, if you switch off the news when presenters begin discussing health-related topics, slowly start watching a few minutes at a time when you are comfortable. Try to do this slowly, as too much, too soon can induce more anxiety.

Breathing exercises, mindfulness and meditation are all good ways to combat any type of anxiety and can help you become a less anxious and stressed-out person in general. If you are not sure where to start with this, you can go online and search for guided meditation videos or try reading books on mindfulness.

Finding professional help when required is absolutely key. If your anxiety is not helped by simple exercises like the ones above, then it is imperative that you speak to your doctor and medical care team, as they should be able to refer you to mental health services for other treatment options such as medication, counselling and therapies such as CBT.

What is the difference between health anxiety and managing my chronic illness?

The behaviours of someone with health anxiety can look very similar to those of someone who is simply managing a chronic illness. The difference between the two is that someone with health anxiety does not necessarily have any illness or disability. A lot of the time their anxiety is surrounding things that could happen, or they are basing their assumptions of ill health around physical symptoms either related to anxiety (headaches, dizziness, heart palpitations) or regular symptoms that many people get from time to time (sore throat or stomach-ache, etc.).

Someone living with a chronic illness, condition or disability (even an undiagnosed one) has regular and measurable symptoms that they experience on a daily basis, such as pain or fatigue. Managing your chronic illness may require you to monitor your health very carefully and it may stop you from doing certain activities. However, the important distinction is that someone with a chronic illness will actually be experiencing a huge variety of symptoms, whereas someone with health anxiety is *worrying* about experiencing a huge variety of symptoms but are not actually experiencing them.

That's not to say, of course, that someone with a chronic illness can't also experience health anxiety about things they don't actually have. Being unwell or disabled full time can make you paranoid about your body, especially if you are struggling with your mental health and see the worst in everything.

> **Reflections**
>
> Have you experienced symptoms of anxiety?
>
> If so, how have they affected your physical health?

2

Medical gaslighting

Medical gaslighting is unfortunately a common occurrence within the spoonie community and we must raise awareness of it in order to stop it. This chapter will outline exactly what medical gaslighting is, who it may affect and what impact it has on those affected.

I have included some tips on how to handle medical gaslighting based on both my own experiences and those of the thousands of spoonies I have met online who have been on the receiving end of this gaslighting, too.

What is medical gaslighting?

Medical gaslighting is a term used to describe the behaviour of medical professionals who invalidate, ignore, dismiss or downplay their patients' symptoms. They may also attribute the patients' physical symptoms to something else, such as a psychological condition, without carrying out any testing or physical examinations.

For example, someone with extremely painful periods may be dismissed by medical professionals who state that all periods are supposed to hurt. Later down the line, this patient may then find they have a chronic illness like endometriosis, which would explain the extreme pain they experience.

What can medical gaslighting sound like?

People from all walks of life can and do experience medical gaslighting and it is important that you know what it looks like so that you can spot it too, if it ever happens to you.

Personally, I've had my own symptoms be dismissed by doctors. I have been told that I simply need to lose weight and then I will no longer be in pain. I have also been informed that women can handle more pain and so I need fewer painkillers than men, and that I need to just learn to live in pain and move on.

Below are some more examples of gaslighting by medical professionals that I have either heard personally or that other spoonies in my community have heard.

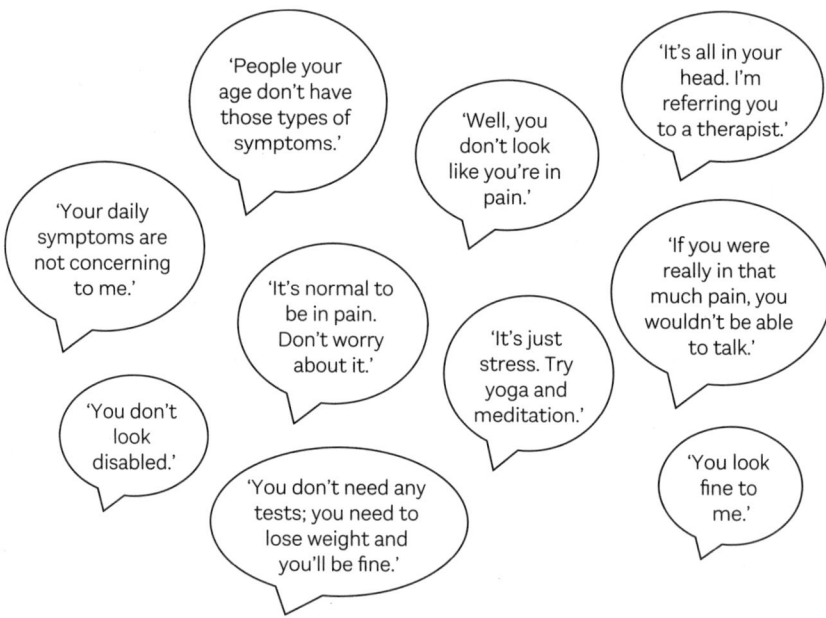

As you can see, phrases like these are used to minimise and deny the realities of the spoonie's experience, and there are even several blatant refusals to refer patients for medical testing. Overall, this medical gaslighting from medical professionals suggests a lack of importance placed on the welfare of the patient.

If you are hearing these types of phrases from your doctor or healthcare professionals, then it may be time to consider making a change. By this I mean you could change your doctor or healthcare facility, get a second opinion, or begin to advocate for yourself and your needs more (see p. 96). Finding a doctor you trust and who will listen to your concerns is a game-changer. If you are unhappy with the medical professionals currently treating you, you are well within your rights to switch to a different one or ask to make your appointments with a specific one within your surgery who you prefer. Although this can be difficult, I've personally found it so much more difficult to live your life not being believed, especially by medical professionals who should know better and should want to help you heal.

Who will experience medical gaslighting?

As someone who has received my own fair share of medical gaslighting (and as someone who speaks to a whole community of spoonies online who has experienced this too), I have now come up with my own personal theory, outlined below.

The 3Fs

1. Female
2. Fat
3. Foreign

I believe that if you fall into one or more of these categories, your chances of being on the receiving end of medical gaslighting are much higher. If you happen to fall into all three categories (as I do) it can seem like medical gaslighting is an unavoidable part of your chronic illness journey. Let's break down what I mean by each of these three Fs.

1. Female

There is a distinct lack of medical data in female bodies in terms of medical science and research. This can lead to female-born patients being misdiagnosed, mistreated or simply having their symptoms ignored and dismissed altogether.

In more recent years this gap in data has begun to be filled, but there is still much more research conducted into the way male bodies behave and how medications and treatments work for male-born patients. The fact that medical professionals are unaware of the way medical conditions can manifest within women can mean that when women describe a laundry list of symptoms, doctors may not know or understand what they are looking at. This is a problem within the entire medical industry, not just with individual doctors, and requires more research, funding and training at all levels of the medical industry, including research, education and practitioners.

Another reason why female patients may be dismissed by their doctors could be plain old misogyny rearing its ugly head. Many medical professionals will dismiss a woman's symptoms as the complaints of an overreacting female. They may be disinclined to believe what a woman is telling them or believe that they are weaker or exaggerating their pain. A survey in 2019 found that 17 per cent of women felt they had been treated differently at the doctor's office due to their gender, while only 6 per cent of men said the same. In the same survey a quarter of women with chronic illnesses said their healthcare provider ignored or dismissed their symptoms and one third said they felt they needed to 'prove' their symptoms. Furthermore, it was found that one in four of these women felt their healthcare provider did not take their pain seriously. While this is self-reported data, it is clear that men did not have the same experiences of being dismissed and ignored in the doctor's office.

This is unacceptable and should not still exist in modern society. Doctors of all genders need to get better at respecting women and their lived experiences, and the medical science industry as a whole needs to plug the gaps in data and research that can allow this type of medical gaslighting to continue to occur.

2. Fat

Overweight patients in the doctor's office are continually dismissed. Their symptoms are often put down to being weight-related, and they are prescribed weight-loss and lifestyle changes without any testing or medical treatments. I have been overweight my entire life and I have personal experience with this in medical settings where I have been ignored and refused testing or physical examination and told to simply lose weight. Unfortunately, this is also a reality for many of the overweight spoonies I have spoken to online.

A study of 4,700 medical students in the USA found that 67 per cent had shown an explicit weight bias and 74 per cent had an implicit weight bias. This means over half were consciously aware that they had negative feelings towards overweight and obese people. It is important to note here that these explicit biases were not unconscious or involuntary: the medical students were aware of having them. As the future of medicine, these people will begin their careers with what they describe as 'negative feelings' towards obese and overweight people. Throughout their careers they will be treating fat people every single day. They will therefore have opportunities to deny care, refuse referrals and dismiss patients. Every. Single. Day. Good luck, fellow fat people...

On a more positive note, I've got your back. We'll circle back to some self-advocacy tips later on, so you can learn how to fight in these types of circumstances (see p. 96).

3. Foreign

I want to start this one by making it clear that my use of the word 'foreign' here simply means 'non-white' and I am using it to make my 3Fs point more memorable and easier to understand.

Medical data has huge gaps in the context of understanding symptoms, conditions and treatments and their effects on Black and Brown bodies. Most research is still carried out on straight white men and applied to all people the same. Unfortunately, this can and does lead to misdiagnoses and the total invalidation of the lived experiences of non-white people.

In 2016 a study found that nearly half of the sample of white medical students believed that Black people had thicker skin than white people. Basic misconceptions like these have also given rise to the incorrect idea that people of colour have greater resistance to pain than white patients. Beliefs like these can be extremely harmful to patients and can also shape the accepted medical practice. These ideas put non-white patients at risk of being misdiagnosed, dismissed or left untreated.

Medical science needs to continue to plug the gaps in data and staff need to train and be taught the real differences and similarities between skin colours. Made-up ideas like a higher pain tolerance in non-white patients has serious consequences.

Reminder: anybody can experience medical gaslighting at the hands of healthcare professionals. Simply because you do not fall into one of these three categories does not mean it cannot also happen to you.

Community column

'I am a fat woman originally from South America and now living in Europe. I agree so much with your [3Fs theory]. I've sadly experienced medical gaslighting many times, even using all three reasons in one appointment. Now every time that I have an appointment I have panic attacks the day(s) before, and I only seek medical advice when it's completely necessary.' – Adriana

'Yep. Totally relate. [I'm] female and my weight fluctuates and [I] have had major issues with medical gaslighting. Definitely avoided doctors – and delayed diagnosis – as a result.' – Mercedes

What is the impact of medical gaslighting?

The impact of medical gaslighting on the patients experiencing it are varied and far-reaching. When patients are on the receiving end of this type of negative treatment from trusted medical professionals it can lead to them losing trust in the professionals and avoiding future medical appointments, which can have a huge impact on their health. If a patient is experiencing symptoms on a daily basis and their own doctor does not believe them – assumes it is a psychological issue and sends them home untested and untreated – it can become difficult for the patient to believe their own mind. They can then go on to develop difficulty in decision-making and believe themselves to be untrustworthy.

The impact of this behaviour can leave behind trauma, which can develop into mental health issues such as depression and anxiety (as discussed on p. 78 and p. 82) and make patients even more vulnerable than they already may be.

This can also lead to self-gaslighting. In table 5, below, I've given examples of what self-gaslighting can sound like, alongside ideas for how we can reframe it into more realistic, positive thoughts.

Table 5 Examples of self-gaslighting and how to reframe it

Self-gaslighting thoughts	Reframing these thoughts
I'm just overreacting.	I'm not overreacting: I'm expressing how it made me feel.
I shouldn't feel like this.	My feelings are my own to feel, no matter what.
I should stop exaggerating; it wasn't that bad.	It's not an exaggeration if it hurt me.
I don't deserve to be happy.	My past mistakes do not define my future.
Maybe it's all in my head.	My experiences are real and valid.
I'm being too sensitive. It's not a big deal.	If it affected me like this, it's an opportunity for me to understand myself better by figuring out why.

A good way to learn to reframe these thoughts is by identifying the self-gaslighting thought pattern within yourself and thinking about how you would respond if someone you love said it about themselves. If your best friend made a negative comment about themself, what would you say in response? What would you want your friend to know, if they were saying these things about their own experiences? Chances are you would be much kinder to your friend than you would be to yourself, and you wouldn't want them to have these types of negative thoughts. Treat yourself how you would treat that friend, and your thoughts about yourself and your experiences will become much kinder and more reasonable.

> **Reflections**
>
> Have you ever experienced medical gaslighting?
>
> How did it make you feel at the time?
>
> How do you feel about it now?

Advocating for yourself

Advocating for yourself is an important part of the spoonie experience, for all the reasons we've discussed above. In a medical setting, where our focus will be here, advocating for yourself can mean remaining firm about any tests, scans or treatments you want your doctor to perform or speaking up when you feel like you are being dismissed.

Learning to advocate for yourself and your needs is a difficult process that can take a lot of practice and is likely to be ongoing throughout your spoonie journey. Sometimes it involves building a thicker skin and gaining the confidence to stand up to a person of authority. Medical professionals have a power over you when you have a chronic illness, as they can either make your life easier or harder. Confronting them when they are making things more difficult for you is essential and – despite it being a hard and sometimes an uncomfortable task – the benefits outweigh the negatives.

As someone who has had to learn these things over many years, trust me when I tell you that sticking up for yourself does get easier with practice and time. Self-advocacy is like a muscle that needs to be built up slowly and strengthened through use, so let's look at how we can do this now. Below is a list of helpful tips for self-advocacy, which we will go through in detail in this section.

1. Do your own research
2. Bring evidence
3. Make a list of questions
4. Keep asking
5. Speak up
6. Bring an ally
7. Make a change
8. Book a double appointment

1. Do your own research

The first step towards being able to advocate for yourself in a medical setting is to do your own research. We live in a world where information is just a click away, and you need to take advantage of that fact. It is crucial that you know everything you can about your symptoms, your illness, your disability and your rights. By doing this, you will be able to ask the right questions and understand what you are being told.

Medical jargon can be a barrier to your care and the fact that busy doctors simply do not have the time to explain everything in great detail can lead to miscommunication and misunderstanding. It is your right to know what is going on with your care, and if doctors are unable or unwilling to provide clarity, you need to seek it elsewhere. Take the time and use the spoons to become an informed patient wherever possible.

Reminder: always use reputable sites for your research and multiple sources wherever possible to ensure you are getting accurate information.

2. Bring evidence

If you have a theory, show some evidence. By tracking your symptoms, side effects, sleep, food and water intake (and anything else you think may be helpful, see p. 33), you can provide your medical team with some evidence that they can refer back to when speaking with you.

Symptom tracking is particularly helpful to have on hand if you have your own theory that you'd like to discuss. For example, if you feel faint throughout the week and believe it may be due to exertion, you could track your blood pressure and pulse rate throughout the day, as well as your activity levels, and see if there is a correlation between the two. Once you can identify a trend or pattern, speak with your care team and discuss treatment options, providing your own data as proof.

3. Make a list of questions

In a short and often rushed appointment it is so easy to become flustered and forget all of your questions. It has happened to me dozens of times: I go into an appointment wanting to discuss five things and immediately forget half of them when I see the doctor. So, for several years, I have been writing a list of questions and discussion topics beforehand and taking it with me. I do this both on paper and on my phone, because though I prefer to have it written on paper, in the past I have forgotten my list (thanks, brain fog!). For this reason I keep a back-up on my phone, in the notes app, to ensure I am still able to discuss everything I need to.

It is perfectly normal to have difficulty recalling everything your doctor says to you, so here are a couple of tips that I have found helpful:

1. Take a pen and paper to every appointment and make notes as the doctor is speaking to ensure you have all of the information you need when you get home.
2. Use your phone to record the whole appointment so you can listen back to it later.

4. Keep asking

This one is pretty self-explanatory. If there is something you want from your doctor or care team (a certain referral, medication or treatment, etc.) ask more than once. Early on in my chronic pain journey I would ask my doctor for various referrals, and he would deny my requests. I eventually stopped asking after being turned down once or twice. To this day, I wish I had kept asking even after being refused. My doctor did not send me to specialists until I had already been in pain for about eight years and by then I had become disabled and begun using mobility aids on a daily basis due to the pain. I often wonder if earlier referrals could have helped in my situation, so I always tell other spoonies to keep asking.

Whether it is testing or new treatment options or different medications, it is so important to let your doctor know what you want and why you think it would be a good fit for you. I will add to this point that if your doctor is giving good reasons why they are refusing a particular request, listen carefully to them and be open to reconsidering your view. For example, if you have back pain and you're requesting a scan of your abdomen your doctor will likely have something to say about why you don't need that.

5. Speak up

You deserve respect, fair treatment and to be heard. This is not up for debate. If you are being treated disrespectfully, or if you feel you are not being heard or feel ignored or mistreated, then I urge you to speak up. Let your doctor know you are unsatisfied with the care they are providing; tell your specialist they need to take the time to explain things more clearly; do not allow anybody to brush you off or treat you like an inconvenience. It is your right to know what is going on with your treatment, understand the procedures being carried out and why. Never accept less than the best for yourself.

6. Bring an ally

Sometimes in a rushed appointment it can be difficult to keep up with everything that is being said, ask all of your questions, remember your doctor's responses *and* advocate for yourself all at once. If you are someone who struggles with these things it is a good idea to bring someone along who can help. A family member, friend or carer can remind you of anything you may forget to ask your doctor, explain any symptoms you may forget to mention, and listen to what the doctor is telling you as well. What's more, they could also think to ask a question you might not have considered and can make suggestions that could help you too. Finally, they may be able to call out medical gaslighting when they see it, witness it for any complaints you may want to file or even greatly reduce the chances of it happening in the first place. It's an unfortunate thing to hear, but sometimes having another person in the room besides the doctor and the patient could mean that the doctor will be less likely to say something insulting, and more likely to listen with empathy. Plus having some back-up is never a bad thing and another person at your appointment means you have someone to sit next to on the bus home.

7. Make a change

Sometimes, even when you have tried all of the above steps, it becomes clear that a particular doctor, nurse, carer or hospital is simply not a good fit. Despite trying to make it work, it can be easier to change doctors or hospitals and find someone or somewhere that works better for you. It can be a difficult decision, but if it is ultimately what is best for you, it is worth the extra effort. Check on your hospital or surgery's website to see how you can go about this process. It will vary depending on where you live.

8. Book a double appointment

A five- or ten-minute appointment with your doctor may not always be enough to discuss everything you need to. Sometimes a double appointment may be necessary. The timings may not always work out due to your doctor's schedule, and you may need to wait slightly longer to find a double slot, but it's always worth asking.

Reminder: you deserve doctors and nurses who listen and believe you, understand your needs and work hard to help you. You deserve a hospital or healthcare facility that has everything you require.

> **Reflections**
>
> Have you ever been gaslighted? How did that make you feel?
>
> How can you implement these self-advocacy tips at your next medical appointment?

3
Distancing yourself from unsupportive people

Being ignored and dismissed by medical professionals who don't know you or care about you on a personal level is one thing. One horrible thing. But to be disbelieved by people around you – people who should know you better than anybody and love you – is much, much worse. If it is something you have experienced or are experiencing, you know the impact it can have on your mental, physical and emotional well-being. It is something I wouldn't wish on anybody.

Finding out the people around you think your illness is fake, or not as bad as you make it sound, or that your symptoms are being played up to get attention is one of the worst parts of living with a chronic illness. I wish I had some perfectly chosen words to get you through that kind of situation, but unfortunately they simply do not exist. It sucks. Full stop.

The only good thing about it is that you can begin to purge those people from your life wherever possible. Their behaviour tells you that they were never true to you from the start, and you should not waste time convincing them you are telling the truth.

My best advice to you is to let them go and move on (if possible, and it isn't always possible if they are a close family member – see below).

Reminder: protecting yourself from the negativity of unsupportive people is a form of self-care.

As someone who is not a trained therapist or mental health professional, everything I write is through the lens of my own experiences and perspective and is not intended to be medical advice. Every scenario is different, and it may be necessary for you to seek professional help in your own life.

Being forced to defend and explain yourself at every turn is a draining way to live, and it may even make your illness worse in the long term. For example, non-believers are unlikely to be receptive to your needs and accommodations and they may attempt to push you past your body's natural limitations, which can eventually lead to a flare-up. In short, the physical toll that spending time with unsupportive and disbelieving people has on your body is enormous.

Coupled with this, the mental toll of being disbelieved by those around you is immense. Being forced to repeat information again and again, debating and arguing will use up your limited energy and cost you more spoons than you have to spare. It is mentally exhausting to be in 'convince' mode every time you see them, like talking to a brick wall and hoping it talks back. Living your life like that is not worth it, trust me when I say this (from experience). I have spent so much time trying to convince people of my own chronic pain and various symptoms. Let those people go, then move on from them. This can be difficult at first, but it is very much worth it in the end.

If cutting people off from your life completely is not something you can do (because realistically it's not always feasible) then taking a step back from their company should always be an option. Never let these doubters drag you into some kind of debate or argument, because they thrive on the fact they're getting to you, and you simply do not have the energy to keep arguing. Instead, disengage, ignore and stop responding, even though that can be hard.

Community column

'Some people you think you know and think they care about you will say they understand and accept your illness but then later they don't understand, say hurtful stuff, and belittle your illness. This makes it hard to open up about your illness. So always believe yourself and don't belittle yourself because of what they said or did.' – Paige

'The reality is that those who you may have thought were your closest friends and relatives, etc., may be the ones in your life that are the most toxic. Just because someone is family does not give them the right to shame or belittle you. And people who may have been very supportive at the beginning are sometimes the ones that are the most unforgiving when you have to cancel on them yet again. It may take a lot to come to terms with it, and we may never understand how others just don't seem to 'get it', but it's reality and is no fault of yours.' – Kimmi

Reminder: it is not your job to convince anybody that what you are saying is the truth. You can teach and educate and raise awareness about your illness and the impact that it has on your life, but if the other person is not open to understanding the information you are sharing, it's a losing game.

Finding community

In a perfect world, everyone around you will believe what you are telling them about your illness, condition or disability, and the impact it has on your daily life. They will ask insightful and thought-provoking questions, and you will have the perfect answers to help them understand your life. But sadly, we don't live in a perfect world.

As discussed above, sometimes people don't believe you. Sometimes people don't understand. Sometimes people don't care to. And that's OK: you'll learn to live with that and distance yourself where possible. But, when it becomes clear that it is time to put some distance between yourself and those who cannot support you, it is vitally important that you do find support elsewhere.

This is because the mental toll of life as a spoonie is huge. So, finding a supportive network is a great way to reduce that toll in some way, whether that is a spoonie community where you can learn more about your illness and share advice or a general community simply as a means to take your mind off your symptoms for a while.

If the idea of doing this sounds daunting to you, then please don't worry. As someone who felt like an outsider for a long time myself, I can guarantee you'll find help and support if you go looking for it in the right places. You can meet new people through:

1. Shared interests
2. Shared experiences
3. Volunteering
4. Online

1. Shared interests

Meeting new people through shared interests is probably one of the easiest ways to find support and community. Join groups dedicated to your hobbies and interests and meet like-minded people either online or in person. Whether it is crafting, music, gaming or pretty much anything else, there's probably a group for it. Use local newspapers, noticeboards or posters at local venues to find groups in your area. You could also look for online groups if you'd prefer to join virtual meet-ups instead. Whether meeting online or in person, remember to be safe and use caution when giving out personal information.

2. Shared experiences

Living with a chronic illness or disability is tough, so finding others with the same kinds of experiences is refreshing. Fortunately, the spoonie community is widespread and diverse and includes some of the best people you will ever know. They may have knowledge or tips for surviving as a spoonie that you haven't come across before, and you can share your own knowledge, too (and recommend a certain book to them . . . wink, wink). Finding these types of people can be done online or in person.

In-person support groups can be illness- or disability-specific or more generalised, and they are often informal. This means you do not need to attend every session or pay a membership fee. This is great for spoonies, as we often don't know how we'll feel on a week-to-week basis. These types of groups may also arrange day trips and visits to local places that can be interesting to members and can help build friendships.

Finding these local support groups is usually fairly easy and can be done by:

- Checking your local government websites for information
- Contacting local charities for any information they may have
- Checking municipal buildings' noticeboards for local groups (hospitals, doctor's office, library, etc.)
- Following your local government social media pages to find information on groups
- Searching social media for key terms like 'disability support' plus the name of your local area or nearest city

3. Volunteering

If volunteering is something you have the time, ability and spare spoons to do then it can be a good way to meet people and make new friends. Local groups may need volunteers throughout the year and would likely welcome the help. These sort of organisations support a wide range of interests, including animal welfare, environmental causes and homelessness, as well as music and performing arts. Finding one that interests you would probably be quite simple, and from there meeting other volunteers or charity organisers is a great way to get to know people with similar values.

4. Online

If meeting new people in person is something you cannot or do not want to do, then meeting people online is a good alternative. Joining shared interest groups online or following social media pages dedicated to things you already like or are thinking about starting can be a great way to meet new people and learn new skills.

There are also plenty of online pages and groups dedicated to living with a chronic illness, condition or disability. This can help you discover people with the same or similar issues as you, so you can share knowledge and advice for surviving as a spoonie. Finding these pages is usually as simple as typing the name of the illness, condition or disability into the search bar and clicking on the accounts related to them. Online spoonie communities can be a huge source of support, so we'll discuss this more next.

Finding community online

When I got my own diagnosis I searched online, via social media, for a place where I belonged. The online spoonie community welcomed me with open arms and words of advice. Yet this is a resource that some medical professionals won't recommend to you; they might not think to tell you that with a few clicks you can connect with people in similar situations.

A simple search will help you find accounts and pages dedicated not only to the general spoonie experience, but to specific illnesses as well. Utilise this resource, as it can and does help so much knowing other people are dealing with similar things as you and have the same illness, condition or disability as you. You can get ideas on how to survive and thrive as well as suggestions for new medications to try or different treatment options that may help you.

With no exaggeration, this community saved my life. It taught me that even though my day-to-day existence looks different now, that does not mean I cannot still achieve what I want. It helped me see that prioritising myself and my health is not only a good thing, but necessary in order to survive. It gave me a place where I truly feel I belong and, in order to pay it forward, I created my own account to help others in the same way, which I have been running for several years.

The idea behind my account (@fourmorespoons) is to help educate, raise awareness and share advice about living with a chronic illness, condition or disability. I share my own journey and continue to learn from my followers, too. It has been one of my biggest and most rewarding challenges, and I love it. My page is a precursor to this book – and is the reason it even exists.

Through the online community I have met so many amazing people from all walks of life, who are either living with their own illness or caring for someone who is. I've also found content creators who share their own journeys, some of which are very similar to my own. I see people thriving with their disabilities and when I first joined, I learned so much in such a short space of time, which helped me manage my daily needs and cope with the idea of living as a young disabled woman.

Creating a spoonie community online

I have named this section of the book 'creating a spoonie community online' because that is exactly what I believe I have done on my own account and I want to help you do the same, if that's something you are interested in. (Quick disclaimer: my community is on Instagram but I've kept my advice general so it can be transferred to most social media platforms.)

Creating my account and community has been hugely beneficial to my overall health and well-being, and I believe I can and have made a difference in many spoonies' lives all over the world. Building this community has made me feel less isolated even when I cannot leave the house, and it gives me a huge sense of satisfaction because I am able to help others and raise awareness all at once. So, in this section, I am sharing some tips and advice for creating your own social media account dedicated to chronic illness and disability content.

Step one

Before starting your account make sure you have a very clear idea of what you want to write about. If you need help working this out, ask yourself these questions:

1. Is there a specific disease/illness/condition/disability you want to talk about?
2. Are there any related topics of discussion to bring up? For example, mental health issues as well as physical health issues.
3. What are you trying to achieve through this account?
   - Education
   - Awareness
   - Fundraising
   - Political change
   - Social change
   - Something else entirely or a combination of all the above
4. What format will your posts take?
   - Short Reel clips
   - Images
   - Long-form videos
5. How much of yourself do you want to show your audience? Will you show your face on camera, for example?

Knowing the answers to these things before you create your account is essential. It means you have an understanding of the way you want your account to look and run, and how you want to connect with your followers.

Step two

Once you have created your account, based on your vision above, the next step is to build a follower base and increase your engagement. In order to do this it is important that you:

- Follow other content creators in your niche. This means you'll have an understanding of what content already exists and helps you decide what you would like to post on your own page.
- Post consistently several times per week to engage with your followers.
- Use hashtags on all of your posts to ensure you are reaching the right audience. It is essential that you are using hashtags relevant to your post and not random ones.

A great tip I got, and still use today, is to create my posts ahead of time, in batches, and pre-write your captions and hashtags. By doing this, you can be more consistent in posting on a regular basis, even when you are especially busy. Personally, at any given time, I have at least one week's worth of posts ready to share to ensure I do not feel rushed in what I am posting. This has helped me immensely in keeping up with the load of work that it takes to create and run a social media account.

Step three

Once you have created an account that you can post to consistently – and that has an engaged following – ask your followers what type of content they would like to see you post. To communicate with your followers you could try the following:

- Create posts that ask specific questions, allowing your followers to answer in the comment section.
- Make it clear that your DMs (direct messages) are open, so your followers know they can message you to ask questions.
- Consider adding your email address to your profile, so people can reach you more easily.
- Try to respond to any comments or questions you receive on your posted content.

If you don't want to be accessible all the time then set up clear 'office hours' and inform your followers that they can message you at any time, but you will be responding only during office hours.

Remember your followers are the community you are catering to, but it is also important that you post things you like and find interesting, so it's good to strike a balance.

Extra tips for creating a chronic illness social media account

- Have a clear, significant and memorable account/username.
- If you decide to use a logo as a display picture, make sure it is easy to understand and recognise, and try not to change it often. You need to ensure your followers recognise your posts in their feed when they see them.
- Creating a brand that is recognisably you is much easier if your content has a colour scheme or format that is kept the same throughout.
- To write and edit your posts, choose an app or program you like and find easy to use. This will depend on the format of your posts; for example, video clips will require a video editing app.
- On each of your posts and all of your content, add a small watermark to let others know it is yours.
- Create posts that include tips for your audience to ensure they are sharing them to their friends and saving them for later. These will boost your engagement and ensure more people are viewing your posts.
- Use your account 'insights' to understand what time your followers are online and active, to know when the best time to post would be.

Reminder: follower counts do not matter; even if your posts only ever reach a handful of people, they can still have a profound impact.

> **Reflections**
>
> If you were to create your own social media account dedicated to chronic illness, what would you name it?
>
> What would you focus on?

4
Imposter syndrome and self-doubt

Imposter syndrome is the feeling of inadequacy that can remain even once a person has evidence of success. These feelings can be experienced in all areas of life, including work, relationships and friendships.

Within the chronic illness and disability context, imposter syndrome is common, and it can manifest as someone feeling like they are faking their own condition, doubting that it is real and questioning their own mind. This can occur even when a person has 'evidence' in the form of medical testing, prescriptions, letters from doctors and lived experiences.

Imposter syndrome in this context can be dangerous because it may lead to spoonies ignoring their own needs and limitations, and therefore poorly managing their illness, condition or disability. This can lead to more frequent flare-ups and more high-symptom days. This further damage may even become permanent, as was the case in my own situation.

Therefore, it is so important, as spoonies, that we fight off the negative self-talk and self-doubt of imposter syndrome and ensure we are carefully and successfully managing our illness, condition or disability in the way that works best for us. Let's explore all of this in more detail now.

Who might experience imposter syndrome?

Anyone can be affected by imposter syndrome at any time. However, within the context of spoonies there are several groups of people who might be more susceptible. These include those who have:

1. Invisible illnesses (*see* p. 30)
2. Dynamic disabilities
3. Experience of being medically gaslit by healthcare professionals (*see* p. 89)
4. Experience of being medically gaslit by loved ones (*see* p. 103)
5. Spoonies without an accurate diagnosis

> **Key term: dynamic disability**
>
> An illness or disability that will fluctuate in severity between a baseline level and a flare-up. Changes can occur frequently or not very often.

1. Invisible illnesses

Illnesses and conditions such as fibromyalgia, endometriosis and chronic fatigue syndrome (CFS) are invisible. This means there is no visible injury or wound and so the patient is viewed from the outside as 'normal'. In these instances, people cannot tell they are disabled or chronically ill just from their outward appearance. This may lead spoonies to doubt whether their own illness is real or not, especially when those around them express some form of doubt too. This type of imposter syndrome can either be a constant worry and presence in the mind of the spoonie or something that just happens from time to time.

2. Dynamic disability

A dynamic disability is a type of disability that can change in severity. This means that symptoms can flare up and worsen from time to time and then return to a 'normal' daily baseline. These shifts can lead to feelings of doubt and confusion, all of which feed into imposter syndrome. A good example of this is seen in ambulatory wheelchair users. This means a person may need a wheelchair sometimes, but not all of the time, as they can walk and move their legs when their symptoms allow them to. In this example, during a flare-up a person may need their wheelchair to get around but once the flare-up is over, and they no longer need a wheelchair for long periods of time, they could begin to doubt whether they really needed it in the first place and to wonder whether they were being dramatic or faking it during their flare-up.

3. People who have been medically gaslit by healthcare professionals

Medical gaslighting is closely linked to imposter syndrome. As previously discussed (see p. 89), medical gaslighting is where medical professionals dismiss, ignore or downplay a person's symptoms and illness, and may refuse referrals or testing as a result of their own biases.

This type of behaviour from a trusted medical professional can add to a spoonie's imposter syndrome. When an authority figure like a doctor – someone who should be dedicated to helping heal us – doubts our experiences it becomes so much easier to question ourselves and our own experiences and recollections. By doubting our truth and lived experiences, medical professionals are opening the door to us beginning to do the same to ourselves.

4. People who have been medically gaslit by loved ones

Medical gaslighting may also occur when our illness is doubted or questioned by those around us, including by loved ones (see p. 103), carers or even strangers. When outside forces undermine our experiences, on top of the doubts cast by medical professionals, it can feel like the questioning is coming from every angle. All of this may lead to a spoonie doubting whether their symptoms are really that bad, and so faking being well to avoid further judgement and eventually causing more flare-ups and high-symptom days due to poor management of their illness, condition or disability. It can be difficult to make sense of your situation and manage it correctly when everyone around you, and sometimes even yourself, is doubting it exists.

5. Spoonies without an accurate diagnosis

When spoonies living with chronic symptoms are pushing for testing and treatment options without an accurate diagnosis it becomes so much easier to fall victim to imposter syndrome. Life with a chronic illness, condition or disability is much easier once you have a name or a word for what you are experiencing. In my case, it took eight years to get a diagnosis and for many spoonies it can take even longer. Once we know what exactly is going on in our bodies it is easier to accept that an illness, condition or disability actually exists.

Ways to fight imposter syndrome

There are several ways to overcome and fight imposter syndrome when it strikes you or those you love:

1. Know the signs
2. Track your illness
3. Reach out for support
4. Be kind to yourself

1. Know the signs

Knowing what to look out for when it comes to imposter syndrome is so important for spoonies, but also for those who care for you. The thought patterns and behaviours attached to imposter syndrome in a spoonie can include dismissing symptoms, overexerting instead of pacing, ignoring doctor's orders, missing appointments and mismanaging your illness, condition or disability. When you stop taking care of yourself or begin to allow yourself to fall behind in managing your illness it can be a clear sign that imposter syndrome may be setting in. Being alert to this and spotting warning signs can enable you to tackle imposter syndrome early on.

2. Track your illness

Providing proof to yourself that your illness and symptoms exist is a major step in fighting off imposter syndrome. Keeping careful records of your illness, symptoms, medications and any side effects (as discussed on p. 33) will give you empirical data to read and absorb when feelings of doubt hit you. This type of first-hand information is invaluable in allowing you to remember that your symptoms may fluctuate but that does not mean your illness, condition or disability is fake.

3. Reach out for support

You are not alone. Other people in the spoonie community can and do have these types of thoughts and feelings. Doubts are natural, especially if you have experienced medical gaslighting from trusted professionals. Reaching out to others in the community can help reassure you that you are not alone. You can do this by joining support groups or online forums, searching for content creators like me (@fourmorespoons) who will validate your experience, or speaking to other people you may know with a chronic illness.

If you are not able to reach out to other spoonies, speak to your loved ones. Family and friends experience your illness or disability too, though in different ways. They observe it from the outside and can see the toll it takes on you. Talk to them about the things they may have witnessed, to combat the self-doubts you may be experiencing. Sometimes viewing yourself from a different perspective can break through the imposter syndrome.

4. Be kind to yourself

Living with a chronic illness, condition or disability is hard enough, so adding self-doubt and feelings of inadequacy is just adding stress to an already stressful situation. Please always remember that you are doing the best you can, so be kind to yourself, because added stress can increase flare-ups and cause more issues in the long run.

Fighting off imposter syndrome is probably one of the only things that is harder than living with an actual chronic illness, condition or disability. When the doubts come from an internal dialogue, rather than from outside, it can be very difficult to fight them off. If people around you doubt your experiences it might be easier to push back and defend yourself against a visible source of negativity, but when the call is coming from inside the house it can be hard to even see or hear the doubts until they are already cemented in your brain and doing long-term damage.

I hope that the tips I've given you in this chapter will help you spot signs of imposter syndrome and give you the tools to combat it.

5

Burnout

Burnout is a state of mental and physical exhaustion that can occur due to prolonged stress. Often this stress is related to work, family and health, but it can include anything that is stressful in your life, including a combination of different things all at once.

Spoonies in particular can be prone to burnout due to the long-term stress of living with and managing a chronic illness, condition or disability. Additionally, those around us helping us to manage our illness or disability can also experience prolonged stress and be vulnerable to burnout. So, it's important to be able to recognise it in ourselves and others.

Signs of burnout

Table 6, below, lists some of the common signs of burnout that you need to be on the lookout for.

Table 6 Common signs of burnout

Drained	Tired	Trapped
Self-doubt	Overwhelmed	Helpless
Procrastination	Insomnia	Run-down
Vulnerable to acute illnesses	Irritability	Impatience

Reminder: managing burnout symptoms can be particularly difficult for spoonies because they can make dealing with your regular symptoms even more difficult.

All of these signs and symptoms of burnout have an overall effect on your physical, mental and emotional health and well-being. There is also significant overlap between chronic illness symptoms and those of burnout, making it difficult to unpick what is causing what. So, let's take a closer look at all of the areas of your life that burnout symptoms can and do have an effect on.

Sleep

Issues with your regular sleep schedule, including disturbed sleep, insomnia, trouble drifting off or trouble staying asleep are all signs of burnout in people with prolonged stress. The overall impact of these sleep issues can compound the impact that burnout has on your body, including issues with managing your chronic illness, condition or disability.

Mood

Low mood, irritation, apathy and mood swings can be signs of burnout, and they can all impact your social life and close relationships in the long term. They also make coping with your chronic illness, condition or disability harder.

Mental health

Depression and anxiety are common signs of burnout if they are new symptoms within the person experiencing it. Mood, sleep and energy level changes can also threaten your mental health and your overall management of your chronic illness, condition or disability.

Energy

Feelings of exhaustion and fatigue can be easily recognisable signs of burnout, especially if they are new symptoms not regularly experienced.

This can make it much more difficult to manage you spoonie symptoms and motivate yourself to take care of yourself or others.

Cognition

Decreased cognition, increased confusion, poor memory and brain fog are all signs you may be experiencing burnout. This can have multiple knock-on effects when it comes to managing your spoonie life, not least managing your medications and attending appointments.

Behaviour

Withdrawal and antisocial behaviour are signs of burnout in people where this behaviour is vastly different from the norm and can have a lasting effect on mental, physical and emotional well-being.

Managing burnout

It can be difficult to manage burnout while experiencing all of these various symptoms. The physical and mental toll can make it hard to muster the will to do anything, let alone deal with what is causing you such additional and prolonged stress.

To help you a little, here are some suggestions for the various ways you could handle it:

1. Track stress
2. Get professional help
3. Find a support network
4. Create work–life balance
5. Prioritise self-care
6. Get adequate, good-quality sleep
7. Ensure you get good nutrition
8. Set boundaries
9. Outsource certain tasks

1. Track stress

Tracking your stress levels can allow you to identify triggers and see patterns of behaviour that can increase your burnout symptoms. This stress tracking can happen alongside symptom tracking – *see* p. 33 for more information. Tracking these things will allow you to eliminate stressors that are causing your burnout symptoms wherever possible. It can also help you determine what needs to change within your life to eliminate the cause of your burnout. The next step is to know what to do when your stress levels are prolonged or increasing – *see* p. 21 for stress-relieving ideas.

2. Get professional help

Seeking professional help from a therapist or coach is a good way to tackle burnout. They are likely able to provide you with techniques to manage and combat stress in your daily life, reducing the chances of you reaching burnout.

3. Find a support network

Having a good support network, including family, friends and carers, if necessary, is essential in reducing your stress and combatting burnout symptoms. Be honest with your loved ones and allow them to help when you need it. Remember, leaning on the people around you is not a weakness, and you would likely not hesitate to help your loved ones if the shoe were on the other foot.

4. Create work–life balance

If work and professional stress is the root cause of your burnout, making adjustments so that you can achieve a decent work–life balance is necessary to manage your burnout. You need to ensure you are not overworking and overexerting yourself at work. A healthier balance between your work and personal life is a good way to manage and reduce your burnout in this type of scenario, though I appreciate this can be hard to do.

5. Prioritise self-care

Regardless of the cause of your burnout, self-care is a must. This can and does look different for everybody. For some it looks like a spa day to decompress and relax; for others it is relaxing with a good book or vegging out on the sofa with your comfort show. Whatever self-care means for you, it is necessary when dealing with burnout to take the time out and do something you enjoy, that brings you some peace and happiness. Self-care is not a one-time thing, though: you must be doing it regularly for it to be effective. Having a day off once every three months is not going to cure you. You need to take time to rest and recover regularly in order to manage and reduce your burnout, even though this can be very difficult if you have dependents.

6. Get adequate, good-quality sleep

Practising good sleep hygiene is essential when dealing with burnout, as well as a chronic illness, condition or disability. Follow these steps for better sleep:

- Cut out caffeine
- Only get into bed when you are ready to sleep
- Avoid screens before bed
- Invest in good-quality bedding
- Get moving during the day
- Get up and go to bed at the same times each day, where possible

7. Ensure you get good nutrition

Ensuring you are eating well and drinking is essential for managing burnout alongside chronic illness or disability (see p. 192 for tips on cooking). You may not feel like cooking and eating nutritious meals every day, but it will help you in the long run. Drinking plenty of water is also a must. Keep a water bottle on hand to make this step easier and if eating a full meal seems impossible, keep healthy snacks nearby to ensure you are eating something.

8. Set boundaries

Depending on the source of your burnout, this will look different for everybody. For instance, if your burnout is rooted in your work, setting strict out-of-office hours is a good example of a boundary that can help. Examine your life in order to identify areas that may be causing burnout. It is then important to ask yourself what boundaries you need to put in place to help with this. Setting and maintaining boundaries can be difficult, but don't worry, there's a section on that coming soon!

9. Outsource certain tasks

Where possible, see if you can outsource some of your tasks to help improve symptoms of burnout. If you have the financial privilege of being able to get paid help for cleaning and other maintenance tasks, that's great, but otherwise reach out to your friends and family to see if they could help. Having someone cook you a meal or take the bins out can help relieve further stress.

See p. 183 and p. 192 for more tips on how to manage cooking and cleaning with a chronic illness, condition or disability.

> **Reflections**
>
> Have you experienced burnout?
>
> How could you use the strategies in this chapter to manage burnout?

Boundaries

It can be difficult to set boundaries, but they are often necessary. As a spoonie it is imperative that you are prioritising your own needs, your health and well-being and protecting your peace. Therefore, setting and maintaining boundaries is not only a good idea, but practically a necessity. As a people pleaser I have struggled with this in the past and honestly, I still do sometimes. Fortunately, for this type of thing, practice makes perfect, but unfortunately nobody can do this for you; you need to do it yourself.

Types of boundaries

Let's start by running through some of the types of boundaries and what they mean:

1. Physical
2. Emotional
3. Time
4. Sexual
5. Intellectual
6. Material

1. Physical

A physical boundary can include a great number of things, including your body, your need for personal space, how comfortable you are with touch, and any physical needs including food, drink and rest. Violations of your physical boundaries can include unwanted touch, having your physical needs denied (e.g. being denied rest when you need it) or having your space invaded.

2. Emotional

Emotional boundaries can include things such as your comfort level with emotional sharing with others, when you share, how much and with whom. Another example of emotional boundaries is deciding your capacity for listening to others and supporting them. It may not be within your capacity at certain times to take on the mental and emotional load of listening to others. Explaining that to them is a type of emotional boundary that it is well within your rights to express. Establishing these boundaries about when you share or when others share with you is essential for everybody.

3. Time

These types of boundaries can include how you spend your time, what your time is worth and how much time you're able or willing to share with others. This can change from day to day. Remember, it is important for you to decide what your time boundaries are and to communicate them with those around you. Time boundaries ensure you are not overcommitting and that you have enough time for all of the various areas of your life. This can be essential for those with chronic illnesses, conditions or disabilities, to ensure they are not pushing themselves too much or too far.

4. Sexual

Sexual boundaries include what you consent to, with whom and when. They also include what you do not consent to. Healthy sexual boundaries require respect, understanding and good communication. It is essential that all involved parties know each other's sexual boundaries, understand any safety rules put in place and know what a withdrawal of consent looks like for all involved parties. Violations of sexual boundaries can include not asking for consent, ignoring a withdrawal of consent, or lying about sexual health, sexual history or contraception use.

5. Intellectual

These types of boundaries can relate to your thoughts, ideas and creativity. This can include how we respond to someone not respecting ideas and suggestions and how we communicate with others and how they may communicate with us. This does not simply mean accepting all thoughts and opinions. It is important for a healthy discussion, debate or discourse to disagree sometimes, especially if what the other person is saying is harmful in some way. A boundary in this instance can be letting the person know you do not tolerate hateful speech, distancing yourself from them or cutting them off completely.

6. Material

A material boundary relates to your possessions, your home and other things you own. Boundaries regarding your possessions include your willingness to share, how much and with whom. These are important boundaries to have, and a violation may look like someone stealing your things or destroying them. It is essential that everyone has and respects these types of boundaries.

How to implement boundaries

When you begin setting boundaries you may feel uncomfortable and guilty for doing so. It can be difficult to start setting boundaries for yourself when you are not used to it, but remember that your needs are important and worth being respected by those around you. Your limitations and how you feel about certain things are worth communicating to those around you in order for your needs to be fulfilled. It is essential that you put yourself first wherever possible (and this can be very difficult if you have children or other dependents, especially if they are also spoonies) and that you can identify what you want and, just as importantly, what you don't want. Looking after yourself and your needs more will help in managing your chronic illness and disability in the long run.

So, how do you set boundaries?

1. Say 'no'
2. Speak up
3. Accept yourself
4. Know your needs

1. Say 'no'

Setting boundaries can be as simple as saying 'no' when people make demands of you that you feel uncomfortable with or are unable to fulfil due to a lack of spoons. Remember that 'no' is a complete sentence and you are not required to justify your denial with reasons or excuses. If something is making you uncomfortable or does not align with your needs or beliefs, it is perfectly acceptable to refuse.

In theory this may be an easy suggestion to make, but in practice you may experience some difficulty, especially if the people you are saying no to are loved ones. Guilt and discomfort are to be expected when refusing to do things, but the only way to get more comfortable doing so is to practise.

2. Speak up

Often, people can, either knowingly or unknowingly, ask too much of us. Whether they intend to do so is irrelevant, though, because if you simply do not have the capacity to do all of the things being asked of you it is essential that you speak up. Ensuring you are not steamrolled by this type of behaviour is a core part of the process of setting boundaries and ending any people pleasing or self-sacrificing tendencies.

This can be a difficult lesson to learn, as it can be distressing to speak out, especially if you are alone against multiple people or someone in a position of authority over you. However, ultimately it is a necessary requirement for setting boundaries and saving your mental and physical energy.

3. Accept yourself

Understanding and communicating your needs is a crucial part of setting boundaries. In order to fully understand your needs and desires and go about fulfilling them, a certain amount of assessment and self-acceptance is required, and you will have to be totally honest about what you can and cannot do in reality. This requires accepting yourself for who you are today, rather than who you once were or who you may become.

If you cannot accept who you are, how can anybody else?

4. Know your needs

Recognising your own needs can be difficult. They may change from day to day or even more frequently. However, having a clear understanding of what you need and want is crucial. If you can ascertain what they are, you can make measured and definitive choices to reach your goals. This can include setting boundaries for yourself and those around you as well as identifying situations that you no longer wish to be in and removing yourself from them.

Knowing and communicating your needs will also help you manage your chronic illness and disability, as they go hand in hand with self-advocacy as well as the pacing techniques that I have discussed throughout this book.

Setting boundaries can be difficult, especially at the beginning, but it is an important step to take wherever possible in order to determine what is and isn't acceptable to you in various situations. It can also help you express your thoughts and feelings in a way that clearly and decisively communicates your needs and promotes better mental and physical health. Understanding and accepting your own needs will give others the opportunity to be more mindful of them, too, and can allow you greater insight into the needs of those around you.

Reminder: boundaries can apply to any areas of your life, wherever you feel they are necessary.

> **Reflections**
>
> Do you set and maintain healthy boundaries within your own life?
>
> How can you do this more successfully?

3

Finances

1. Loss of income — 135
2. Hidden costs of spoonie life — 143
3. Education and employment — 149
4. Health scams — 157

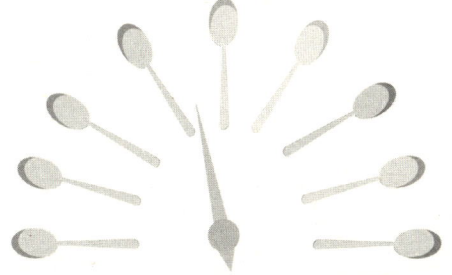

1
Loss of income

As someone with a chronic illness, condition or disability, working an everyday, nine-to-five job can be difficult. Many spoonies are able to do this, usually with some adjustments and accommodations, but for lots of us, working every day is simply not feasible. This is because daily symptoms, unpredictable flare-ups and regular medical appointments mean we may need to take more time off work than we would be able to come in for. As I explain below, we do not all have the same 24 hours in a day. This can lead to a loss of earning potential, which can impact more than just your bank balance.

Lost earning potential

Most people grow up thinking about what their life will look like when they are an adult: what job they will have, the kind of house they will buy and an idea of the lifestyle they want. Unfortunately, a chronic illness, condition or disability can throw a spanner into those plans, very quickly.

Personally, I went to university, got an undergraduate and master's degree and by the time I had graduated I was physically disabled due to my, then undiagnosed, chronic illness. I was never able to use my degrees in a 'real' job because I was physically unable to cope. Growing up, I had wanted a life that included a good job, a nice house and a decent salary that would enable me to look after my parents. I'm not able to have that.

For me, working a nine-to-five job is virtually impossible. Every day I have pain, fatigue and brain fog as well as about a hundred other symptoms. Additionally, I have about three or four medical appointments a month that each take time and energy to attend. I spend my days pacing (see p. 63) to ensure I do not overextend myself and push myself into a flare-up and honestly, some days I still push myself too far, even without a job.

This lost earning potential can be challenging to talk about with friends and family without wallowing in self-pity. It can be complicated because it's a painful reminder that our lives will likely always look different to theirs, and unless they experience it for themselves, they truly cannot relate to you. Nobody who is disabled or chronically ill wants to be in a position where they cannot work and are forced to rely on government benefits or the kindness of their family and friends to survive.

The situation can bring with it a sense of loss for the life you wanted to lead and envisioned you would have. At the same time it can be frustrating and difficult to see your friends and family achieving the types of things you want but simply cannot achieve. Watching friends the same age as you find their career paths, get married, buy homes and thrive is a bittersweet feeling. You can be so proud of their victories, to see them growing, learning and striving to better themselves, but at the same time it can be a challenge to feel like you can only cheer from the sidelines.

This is a tough situation because the last thing you want to do is make them feel guilty for thriving while you feel you are simply surviving. It is nobody's fault, including your own, that you are unable to reach certain goals.

However, while the loss of earning potential is certainly a setback, it doesn't have to be the end of the world. It just means you can and need to create new goals you wish to reach in the future.

> **Reflections**
>
> How would you discuss the financial impact of chronic illness or disability with your loved ones?
>
> Can you reframe the situation and view it as an opportunity to create new goals based on your current reality?

Usable hours

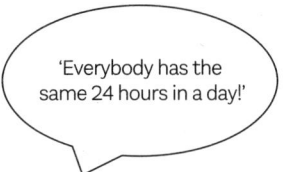

'Everybody has the same 24 hours in a day!'

You've probably heard this saying lots of times in your life. I know I have. But the truth is: no, we don't all have the same 24 hours in a day.

Living with a chronic illness is exhausting and unpredictable. Our bodies can change from one moment to the next; it is impossible to know if we will wake up in pain or well rested, if we will be at our baseline level of symptoms or be experiencing a flare-up. We cannot predict our flare-ups and our good days and most of the time it's blind luck when we are in slightly less pain today than yesterday. Living a life of constant vigilance is draining. We need to be on guard to ensure we are pacing, resting and managing our illness or disability and taking our medications, and about a hundred different things that most people do not need to think about.

Being in pain or incapacitated in some way by disability all day, every day with no breaks, no time off, no holiday, is exhausting. So, no, we do not all have the same 24 hours in a day.

Community column

'I find usable hours vary according to the time of day, weather, the actual type of activity and which symptoms/conditions are taking precedence ... sounds complicated, and it is.' – Ann

'I spend my days hoping that the new symptoms I'm experiencing are not some new illnesses and that they will go away soon. I spend my days researching new treatments and reading medical journal articles, trying to decipher jargon to see if there is some new medication that could help me. I spend my days resting to ensure I can make it to all of my medical appointments this week. We do not have the same 24 hours in a day.' – Anonymous

When it comes to the number of usable hours in a day, this is different for every spoonie. Usable hours are exactly what they sound like: how many hours in the day are available for you to be productive. This can vary from day to day and person to person. On average a healthy, able-bodied person has around 10–14 usable hours in their day. This is time spent running errands, working, doing hobbies, exercising and anything else they want or need to do. A reduction in these usable hours has an obvious impact on spoonies' working lives. Less time to work leads to a direct loss of income. Chronically ill and disabled people generally have far fewer usable hours in a day and so are able to accomplish much less, and need to rest more.

Personally, I usually have around four or five usable hours in an average day, although this does vary depending on my food, drink and medication intake as well as other factors like my sleep, and my usable hours usually require rests and naps in between. It has taken me many years of trial and error to understand how many hours in a day on average I have to carry out the tasks I need to do. I have accepted this about myself and plan my life accordingly. I know that I have the most energy immediately after waking up, so I try to schedule all important appointments for morning slots. When I have errands to run they are always in the morning, and if I have plans to socialise I try to arrange them for as early in the day as possible. By the afternoon I am usually tired and need to rest, and by the evening I am usually too exhausted to function. Errands are done in short bursts and spread out over several days or even a week (and sometimes longer) to avoid overexertion. I also try to squeeze in my hobbies where possible and I continue to rest throughout the day to ensure I am not overdoing it.

In order to successfully manage your own illness, it is imperative that you reflect on your own energy levels and usable hours. This will allow you to figure out a routine that works best for you and your needs. Your usable hours will look vastly different to those of your able-bodied friends and family, but remind yourself that you are not trying to do the same amount of things in the same amount of time. If you are trying to squeeze ten hours of errands and activities into only four hours of your day, of course you will either fail or burn yourself out. The lifestyle section (from p. 167) will go into more details about simple ways in which you can adapt your life to make the most of your usable hours.

How many usable hours do I have?

Figuring out the number of usable hours you have in a day can be difficult, mostly because there is no hard-and-fast rule on how to go about this. When living with a chronic illness or disability energy is often limited and it's possible you may have very few usable hours.

Factors to consider when you are calculating the number of usable hours you have include:

1. Specific illness
2. Symptom intensity
3. Individual needs
4. Type of activity

1. Specific illness

Some chronic illnesses and conditions limit energy more than others. For example, someone living with Chronic Fatigue Syndrome (CFS) will likely have less energy and more fatigue than someone living with type 2 diabetes. While both conditions can cause fatigue, diabetes-related fatigue can be managed with lifestyle changes and better control of blood sugar, while CFS-related fatigue is more persistent and resistant to treatment. Both are chronic illnesses and need their own management strategies and both impact the person's life, and I am certainly not saying one is better or worse than the other, but they do have different symptoms. The point here is that the type of illness you may be living with will have an effect on the number of usable hours you have in a day and is the first factor to consider.

2. Symptom intensity

Symptom intensity can and does change regularly: it can fluctuate from day to day or even minute to minute. It is also highly variable and affects everyone differently. It is a core consideration, since the intensity of your symptoms will have a direct impact on the number of usable hours you have in a day. Think of the difference between your baseline symptoms and your flare-up symptoms (see p. 16). On these days you will likely have very different energy levels and therefore a different number of usable hours.

3. Individual needs

An individual's needs can drastically alter the number of usable hours in a day. Even something as basic as age can alter your needs and therefore the number of usable hours available to you. Someone with the exact same illness or disability, symptoms and intensity of symptoms can require a very different level of pacing and rest than you. Only you can assess your personal needs. This will likely involve a lot of trial and error where you spend more spoons than you should many times before you truly learn what you need. This is very common in the spoonie community and is something that is virtually unavoidable as you try to strike a decent balance between resting and productivity.

4. Type of activity

Certain types of activity cost us more energy than others. In table 1 on p. 6 I listed some everyday activities and the number of spoons they might cost. This is an example of how the type of activity you are engaging in can affect your usable hours in a day. For instance, socialising with loved ones is a strenuous and energy-costing activity that can drain your spoon count very quickly, so you may only be able to do that for an hour at a time. Housework can be a more or less solo activity that may not drain your energy as fast, meaning you may be able to do this for two hours.

Given all these factors, accurately assessing the number of usable hours you have can be difficult. However, it is important that you keep trying. It may take some guesswork at the beginning but eventually you can learn from past experiences and begin to do it more easily, especially if you keep a symptom diary (see p. 35) and note down any triggers or especially spoon-heavy activities.

> **Reflections**
>
> What factors impact the number of usable hours you have on any given day?
>
> Can you identify which specific activities cost you the most spoons and take up a lot of your usable hours?

2
Hidden costs of spoonie life

In addition to the fact that many spoonies are unable to work at all or have to significantly reduce their hours compared to their able-bodied peers, there is a huge variety of hidden and additional costs associated with life with a chronic illness, condition or disability. This is an often overlooked and underacknowledged part of what life as a spoonie looks like and so it is important to highlight it here, to raise awareness and prompt open discussion of these matters. Knowledge is power, after all, and if you know what the costs are, you can at least be mentally prepared for them and take steps to avoid being caught off guard.

Some of these additional and often hidden costs are:

1. Medications
2. Treatments
3. Mobility aids
4. Specialist equipment
5. Shipping and delivery fees
6. Transport fees
7. Specialist dietary requirements
8. Energy and water
9. Insurance
10. Alternative remedies

Let's now look at each in turn. It might be worth making a note of the costs of each category in your own life as you go, so you have the information in front of you and can make an accurate assessment of what your spoonie overheads actually are.

1. Medications

Depending on your location, the cost of necessary medications for your chronic illness, condition or disability can be extremely high. Health insurance may cover some of it and government help may also be available, but generally speaking the cost of prescription medications can be difficult to keep up with. People who require more than one prescription will struggle more, and despite additional assistance they may ignore medical advice by skipping some medication to save on money. This issue is one that many spoonies face in various parts of the world.

2. Treatments

Paying out of pocket for various treatments, such as medical procedures and surgical operations, can get very expensive very quickly. Private treatments may be necessary where public hospitals are at capacity and waitlist times are growing ever longer. When a person is suffering for weeks, months and years on end waiting for treatment, paying privately for (often expensive) treatments can seem like the only option. Medical insurance can be tricky to navigate and use for pre-existing conditions and costs get extremely high when spoonies are forced to pay out of pocket.

3. Mobility aids

It may surprise able-bodied people to know that mobility aids are rarely given to patients for free. When they are, the hospital-issue aids like crutches, walking sticks and walkers are ill-fitted to the patient and not usually suited to individual needs or long-term use. Many spoonies require more specialist aids (*see* p. 180) and often we pay out of pocket for them in order to improve our mobility and to reduce the risk of doing more damage to ourselves in the long run.

4. Specialist equipment

Specialist equipment can include anything from shower chairs and hygiene products to kitchen gadgets to make daily living easier. These are usually paid for by patients, although sometimes government grants and charitable funding may be available to cover a portion of your needs, so it is worth checking if this is an option. Overall, though, it is unlikely that you will get everything you need for free, especially if you need it quickly.

5. Shipping and delivery fees

One thing able-bodied people do not think about is the fact that many spoonies are unable to go out and get everything they need. Online shopping and doorstep delivery is virtually a necessity. This can be an additional cost, as there is sometimes a shipping and handling fee of some kind, and the online grocery price may be higher than the in-store price.

6. Transport fees

Transport fees and additional travel expenses add up when you live with a chronic illness, condition or disability. Sometimes medical appointments are in hospitals or clinics that are too far for public transport, and we may need to get a cab instead. This has happened to me multiple times and trust me when I tell you, it all adds up. When you are constantly exhausted and in pain, deciding between three hours on two buses or a 50-minute taxi ride can be an easy (and expensive) decision to make.

7. Specialist dietary requirements

For many living with a chronic illness, food intolerances and allergies are part of the territory. This can mean that expensive alternatives are not a luxury but a necessity. While it may be easier to find gluten-free or vegan options these days, the prices of these items are still sometimes much higher than their regular counterparts.

8. Energy and water

With a cost-of-living crisis currently happening in many parts of the world, and increasing energy and water bills for everyone, this is something that many people will be worried about. However, for people living with a disability or illness, putting the heating on is not optional. The cold can make joint and muscle pain worse and lead to stiffness and flare-ups. Hot showers and baths can help soothe these aches and pains somewhat and devices like heating pads, hot water bottles and massage guns all help, but they also use up energy and water and cost money. Having the heating or air-conditioning on is also expensive, but often necessary.

9. Insurance

Pre-existing conditions can mean that insurance can be more expensive for spoonies than for able-bodied people. This includes health insurance, life insurance, travel insurance and even car insurance.

10. Alternative remedies

'You should try yoga!' 'You should see my chiropractor!' 'Have you tried acupressure?' 'I heard about this thing. . .'. The list of alternative remedies, health supplements, different diets and must-have devices to help with spoonies' daily symptoms is endless, and they all cost money. Finding alternative remedies is not something that has worked for me personally, and I've tried some really weird things, but if you want to research them and try them yourself, bear in mind the extra outlay they will require.

Unfortunately for many spoonies, the cost of all of the additional items and services listed above can be too high and things we may need can be outside of our budget. This is very stressful, which can make some illnesses worse, and can even lead to debt and other financial strife. Even if we can just about afford them, often all disposable income is spent on necessities, and we no longer have money left over for anything else. Things like hobbies and socialising become less important when you are struggling to pay for insurance or medications that you require to live. This in turn can lead to issues like social isolation (see p. 169) and mental health problems (see p. 77), which make managing a chronic illness or disability so much more difficult.

Managing the hidden costs of spoonie life

I am not an expert in finances, but I suggest that if money is becoming a worry it would be a good idea to research any financial assistance that may be available to you in your area. The list below highlights some of the places where you might find the help and support you are entitled to:

- Local government schemes
- National government benefits
- Local charities that offer assistance
- Charities specifically related to your illness, condition or disability

You can also ask your doctor for help with pointing you to the relevant services, or you might consider reaching out to family and friends. Even if you feel uncomfortable talking about money, discussing your concerns may ease your worries and they may be able to help with your financial planning in ways you may not have thought of. Keeping these concerns bottled up can lead to issues like mental health problems, which will inevitably make managing your chronic illness, condition or disability that much more difficult.

So, although I don't have all, or even any, of the answers, I do recommend that you reach out to the support around you and share your financial concerns wherever possible.

Reflections

Have you been able to accurately assess how much you are having to spend on spoonie-specific expenses?

Can you think of any other hidden costs of spoonie life? Write them down and add them to the other costs, so you have a clear picture of what you are spending.

3
Education and employment

Inaccessibility in education and employment is a huge contributing factor in why many chronically ill and disabled individuals are financially disadvantaged. This is a widespread concern that has huge and far-reaching implications in many parts of the world, so it's important to bring awareness to it here and discuss what can be done.

Accessibility in education

Education often has a direct impact on future earnings, yet many institutions are simply not suitable or accessible for people living with chronic illnesses, conditions or disabilities. By accessibility, I do not just mean ramps or mobility aids; in the education sector, accessibility can mean a range of different things, some of which – such as the three key approaches listed below – are fairly simple to implement.

1. Embrace technology
2. Support diverse learning styles
3. Engage in open communication

1. Embrace technology

Technology in schools can be viewed as a negative or positive thing, but like it or not, it is going nowhere soon. Assistive technologies such as tape recorders, screen magnifiers, text-to-speech software and word prediction are all essentials for disabled and chronically ill learners, and these types of technology should be embraced by educational institutions with disabled students, to allow them to remain in school. Schools should make it clear that this technology is available to all those who need it and all students should be taught how to use it and why it is necessary. This helps to normalise the technology when it is used in the classroom and helps able-bodied students, too, since they may one day need it themselves.

Furthermore, staff should be required to undergo some form of training to ensure they are familiar with this assistive technology, so they can troubleshoot basic issues more quickly and also be familiar with the benefits and limitations so they can recommend it to their spoonie students, if it would be helpful.

2. Support diverse learning styles

There are several different types of learning styles that students will fall into. Not every student will learn in the same way or at the same speed as others and these differences should be supported by teaching staff and the wider institution as much as possible, from nursery right through to further education. This will allow for better outcomes for not only disabled and chronically ill students, but for all students. These different learning styles include:

- Visual: these learners prefer images over text to convey information.
- Auditory: these learners work well with speaking and listening and thrive in situations such as group discussions and lectures.
- Reading and writing: students who learn best through words prefer to translate concepts into words or essays and work well with notetaking and reading.

- Kinaesthetic: these students learn through tactile representations. They are hands-on learners and figure things out by touch.

3. Engage in open communication

This is an essential step for ensuring chronically ill and disabled students are achieving their maximum potential. Students, teachers and administrators should be able to openly discuss the best approaches to learning, the access needs of the students and all relevant information that will help the students learn. Students should feel comfortable pointing out things that they need, and staff should be open to listening to these suggestions.

Students' access needs can cover a huge range of requirements, including but not limited to:

- Ramps and step-free access
- Disabled toilets with additional space, grab rails and an emergency cord
- Clear signage around the institution, including high-contrast colours, Braille and hearing loop options
- Video captions for any footage shown in the classroom or at assemblies and graduations
- Lesson transcripts to ensure students are able to understand the lesson
- A discussion as to whether a print textbook or e-textbook is preferred, or even both

Students taking exams throughout the year require several different adjustments in order to ensure they can perform their best, too. These include, among other things:

- Extra time for exams and assessments
- Breaks throughout the examination session
- A reader to read questions and ensure they can understand them

- A scribe to write answers on the page and ensure they have filled out the paperwork correctly
- Assistive technology such as speech-to-text or a magnifier for students with visual impairments
- A separate room to ensure their needs are being met and there is no disruption to other students

Accessibility in the workplace

Ensuring that workplaces have appropriate accessibility levels is something that is commonly required by law in many countries. However, despite this being a ratified issue, spoonies often find their places of employment are not meeting their access needs and therefore they cannot work there any more. This is a major concern, as it obviously has a huge financial impact and can lead to additional stress and mental health issues, which all have a knock-on effect on the management of a chronic illness, condition or disability.

Accessibility in the workplace should begin within the actual job posting and follow through to the interview and hiring process. Job postings should include details of the job role, detailed information about the required duties and accurate information on the salary expectations and working hours. This information is a requirement for people with chronic illnesses and disabilities and should be standard operating procedure for all job listings, as it could benefit not only spoonies but everybody else, too. Unfortunately, this is not always how things play out – employers often change the title, roles and salary depending on the applicant's previous experience and age, as well as several other factors.

Throughout the interview process accessibility should be made a priority to ensure that disabled and chronically ill applicants are able and willing to apply for these jobs. Access needs for job interviews include, but are most certainly not limited to:

- Ramps and step-free access to the place of employment as well as the interview room and any areas that the applicant will be shown

- Disabled toilets, including additional space for mobility aids, grab rails and an emergency cord
- Clear and easy-to-understand signage in high-contrast colours, with Braille, multi-language and hearing loop functions also available
- Online interviews via video webchat as an option
- A communications support worker should also be allowed to attend the interview at the interviewee's request. This can include a sign language interpreter or lip speaker if required

Once a job offer is made, accommodations and accessibility requirements should be discussed in full between the employee and the employer, with a member of the human resources department present as well, and a support worker for the employee if they request one. This will ensure that all parties are held accountable as well as being heard and respected.

Once an interviewee becomes an employee, access needs can include adjustments such as:

- Ramps and step-free access
- Disabled toilets
- Clear signage
- Flexible working options, including adjusted start and end times and work-from-home options
- Meetings and training courses should be held with in-person and online options to ensure that staff can attend in the way that works best for them
- Specialist equipment that may be required should be purchased and installed; this could include things like assistive software for computers or adapted keyboards and ergonomic office furniture
- All staff, not just those with chronic illnesses, conditions and disabilities, should have easy access to mental health support should they want it

These types of accommodations are important for ensuring that chronically ill and disabled people can remain in the workforce for as long as they would like to. Without these types of accessibility requirements employees are more likely to fall short of targets and be penalised in the workplace.

How to advocate for accessibility

Whether it is in the workplace or an educational institution, advocating for accessibility for yourself and others can be a difficult and arduous process. This can make it seem daunting but the benefits of actually getting what you need to succeed far outweigh the spoons required to make it happen.

Let's discuss some practical tips for how to successfully advocate for yourself and others:

1. Know your rights
2. Know what you need
3. Know how to fight

1. Know your rights

Knowing your rights and what you are entitled to will make it easier for you to advocate for what it is you need. If, for example, you are aware that your right to accessibility is protected by law, and how, this can make it easier for you to request accessibility accommodations from your educational institution or workplace. Depending on where you live, laws and rights may be different, so it is worth doing some research online. Search your location and key terms such as 'disabled access' and phrases such as 'workplace' or 'education' to find out what exactly you are entitled to in your country or state.

2. Know what you need

This may seem like an obvious one, but you need an idea of exactly what it is you require from your school or employer. Every spoonie's access needs will be different and they may even change frequently. Your employer giving you step-free access when what you really need is to work from home is not very helpful. Pinpoint what you need to succeed at work or school and firmly make your case, using your research about your rights to back you up.

3. Know how to fight

I truly hope that when requesting accommodations and accessibility you get exactly what you need with very little fuss. However, as we don't live in a perfect world, this may not always be the case. The final tip I can give you is to be aware of how to fight for your rights. If requests are denied, you need to know what your next steps will be, whether that is an appeals process, some form of tribunal or even legal proceedings. Educate yourself about what any complaints or appeals process may look like. Be firm but respectful when you explain that you are prepared to move forward with these processes and get what you need to succeed, as is your right.

> **Reflections**
>
> Have you ever needed to advocate for accessibility in education or employment?
>
> How did you manage to do this?
>
> What would you do differently another time?

4
Health scams

This chapter will highlight the problem with health scams and how best we can avoid them. As scams are becoming increasingly sophisticated, even spoonies with years of experience can find themselves falling victim to them, so it's important we all know and share as much information about them as possible, to protect ourselves.

What are health scams?

Fraudsters will sell you miracle cures for all kinds of illnesses or disabilities online and in person and, unfortunately, some spoonies will waste their time and money on them. Often, a fraudster will target vulnerable and desperate people in the hope of taking their money and personal information to sell on later. Scammers are adept at taking advantage of your optimism. It may sound cynical to say this but when a person is hopeful about trying new treatments or alternative remedies, they become an easier target for unscrupulous criminals.

Scammers will claim just about anything to try to lure in customers to buy their products. These can be in the form of pills, powders, lotions, devices or even courses. Appearing sympathetic and trustworthy is a skill these criminals excel at employing against their targets. Even experienced consumers are susceptible to these scams, and falling victim to them is nothing to be embarrassed about. I personally have bought all kinds of supplements and devices in the vague hope they would help treat or relieve at least some of my pain and symptoms.

Flyers and posters put up on hospital noticeboards without permission or sellers creating fake profiles online to target vulnerable individuals are both common tactics used to target either those living with the illness or disability themselves, or those who know and love someone who is. Scammers will sometimes sell products that are never actually received, or they may send out fake or useless items.

It is important to remember that many of the diseases and illnesses that these scammers are attempting to target are ones that require individualised treatments on multiple fronts or that simply do not have a cure to begin with. Many of these 'miracle' cures are unresearched, unregulated and could cause you more harm in the long run. So, what are some common ones, and how do you sidestep them? Let's take a look.

Common health and well-being scams

In order to better protect yourself and your money from these scams you need to know what they may look like and what they may be trying to sell you. Scammers make billions of dollars per year from selling fake or misleading products, which include:

1. Cancer cures
2. Chronic pain treatments
3. Diabetes cures
4. Anti-ageing products
5. Vitamins and supplements
6. Addiction treatments
7. Arthritis treatments

Safety warning

Always get your medical advice from trusted professionals and be sceptical about anyone selling a non-prescription cure. Some of these fake medications could be simply placebos, but some may actually cause damage or do harm to you; just because you do not need a prescription for them does not mean they are safe to take. What's more, unproven products can be dangerous as they may interfere with or limit the effectiveness of your prescription medications. If you are unsure of whether a specific treatment or remedy is legitimate or helpful to you, speak with your medical care team to ensure you are not doing yourself more harm. Remember to remain sceptical and listen to your gut when something sounds too good to be true.

Prescription v non-prescription treatments

A prescribed treatment is studied, tested and researched thoroughly by medical professionals and scientists and side effects are tracked and examined in order to improve the product for all those who are taking it. They are rigorously regulated and undergo many safety checks before they are made available for sale.

Unresearched and unregulated products are sold without any of these safety measures in place, so there is no consumer protection.

1. Cancer cures

Scammers will take advantage of the anxiety and worry surrounding a cancer diagnosis to steal your money and information. Miracle pills, powders and herbs are sold to desperate people willing to try anything, but please note that no single remedy can treat a broad range of cancer types. Cancer is a very individualised disease and even two people with the same type and stage of cancer may need two different treatments. Get your information from reliable sources, such as your own medical team or peer-reviewed medical studies, not social media or untrustworthy websites, to avoid losing money and hope to these scammers.

2. Chronic pain treatments

Pain has many different sources: it can be caused by hundreds of different things and sometimes there is no known cause. Pain is also different for everybody who experiences it and so the approach used to fight it must also be different for everybody. A single remedy is unlikely to work, as pain needs to be tackled on multiple fronts. So, a single miracle cure that promises to heal a huge range of things is clearly a scam and should be avoided, even when it is accompanied by testimonials from 'customers' and 'medical experts'.

3. Diabetes cures

There is no known cure for type 1 diabetes; insulin medication and monitoring of glucose and ketone levels are the management techniques used. Type 2 diabetes can be reversed in many people through sustained weight loss and healthy lifestyle choices, but there isn't a quick fix. Scammers selling a miracle drug or service that will immediately cure an illness is a massive red flag.

4. Anti-ageing products

Maybe one day a product will exist that can slow or even reverse the ageing process but right now, this simply does not exist. Pills, devices and lotions designed to target your insecurities surrounding ageing are dangerous. Untested and unregulated products could cause you harm in the worst-case scenario, or in the best-case scenario they do absolutely nothing. The risk that comes with these items is simply not worth it.

5. Vitamins and supplements

There are various health benefits associated with taking vitamins and supplements. They can boost your immune system or help with better sleep, and probably a hundred other different things, too. However, they are not going to cure your illness, condition or disease. Supplements in particular are unregulated and so companies are able to make outlandish claims about their effectiveness without needing to provide any evidence to support them. This means that even if the packaging says that they treat various illnesses and they are being sold by reputable websites, you should still take the adverts with a pinch of salt.

6. Addiction treatments

Addiction is a complicated thing: it is a mix of genetics, social and economic factors as well as physical health, and there is no cure. Treatment requires a multi-faceted approach that is ongoing for years to come, usually including medication, counselling and group support. It is something that needs to be worked on throughout the person's life to avoid relapses or setbacks.

7. Arthritis treatments

Due to the fact that some arthritis symptoms can come and go, it can be easy to assume that a single non-prescription treatment or cure has worked. If the symptoms disappear or ease somewhat after taking a specific remedy, of course you will assume it is because of that product. In actual fact there is no cure for arthritis, there are simply management techniques. Unregulated and unresearched pills or lotions can cause more harm than good and should be disregarded entirely.

How to spot a health and well-being scam

Knowing the tactics that criminals use regularly to attempt to con their customers is an important step in learning to spot a scam when you see it. As consumers have grown smarter and more wised-up about the scammers' techniques, so have the criminals.

Here are some of the things that mark out a health and well-being scam, either online or in person:

1. Outrageous claims
2. Inclusion of false testimonials
3. Money-back guarantees
4. Sense of urgency
5. Use of pseudoscience

1. Outrageous claims

Products with outrageous and exaggerated claims of the types of things they can do should be avoided. A single product that claims to cure a huge variety of illnesses and diseases is clearly fake and you should be wary of using it. A single course or device is unlikely to cure ten different and often unrelated diseases, for example. The makers are simply including a wide variety of symptoms or illnesses in order to con as many people as possible.

2. Inclusion of false testimonials

Legitimate products, devices or courses will often have testimonials from past users or even medical professionals. Scammers are aware that it is easier to trust something when a human face is put on the front of it. Therefore they use false testimonials to try to sell products that are either fake or dangerous, in an attempt to draw in customers. These testimonials can be from fake customers who used their product and loved it or from fake medical professionals explaining the product and its benefits.

3. Money-back guarantees

'Love this product or your money back!' 'Sixty-day money-back guarantee if you buy this product and don't love it!' These types of selling gimmicks are excellent for luring customers in. People see them and assume they will be able to try the product with no or very little risk. Unfortunately, customers then buy the product and find out it doesn't work. When they attempt to get their money back they are usually unable to do so, or the company is no longer in business by the time they are ready to return the product.

4. Sense of urgency

Adverts that instil a sense of urgency in their customers are an effective selling tactic. Often people will purchase something they are not even sure they want if there is a chance they might miss out on some kind of deal. This is compounded when the message is coupled with a money-back guarantee.

5. Use of pseudoscience

Use of phony scientific evidence or terminology can make products appear genuine. As the average person may not know much about science and medicine, throwing in some jargon can add to the appearance of realism and validity. Usually a simple google will show that the words being used in these types of adverts are typically nonsense or being applied incorrectly.

Doing your own research is also an excellent way to check if the actual science behind the product is real. You do not need a scientific degree to use the internet to fact-check a product. If you are not confident in your ability to do this, request help from a loved one or carer or ask a trusted medical professional to explain the science to you.

Community column

'Health scams make me want to scream. It's essentially robbing vulnerable people who are often at breaking point and are looking for help. People who commit these kinds of scamming techniques deserve a special place in hell.' – Laura

> 'If a miracle cure for something existed, we would ALL be telling each other about it for FREE!' – Kathryn
>
> 'I fell for the whole vitamin thing years ago – bought a book that said you could take all these vitamins, minerals, amino acids, etc. and you would get better. Followed the regimen for six months . . . no improvement. These days I have a very highly developed quackometer. Some of the offenders in this regard are actually doctors and that lends some credibility to the ads . . . but actually it means nothing.' – Lorna

How to avoid health and well-being scams

Now that you know some of the various techniques that scammers may use to take your money and personal data, we can discuss a few ways to avoid fake products, devices or courses that are sold online or in person:

1. Do independent research
2. Speak to a trusted professional
3. Improve your online literacy

1. Do independent research

Usually a quick internet search will tell you that there is no cure for type 1 diabetes or any of the other diseases that a single pill claims to cure. Even if you are desperate for relief from your own disease, or are searching to help a loved one, wasting time, energy, money and hope on a fake treatment or remedy will likely do more harm overall.

In order to ensure you are getting an accurate view of the product you are considering, try researching the name of the product or company that is selling it to you and adding words such as 'review', 'complaint', 'scam' or 'lawsuit' to your search. This will ensure you are seeing the most accurate information on the product and that you are aware of the real experiences of past customers, not the fake customer testimonials from scammers trying to sell their product to vulnerable people. If many people are saying it is a scam or that it does not work, or if the makers are currently being sued for selling these fake items, it will be clear that you should avoid the product, service or company altogether.

When deciding on an alternative remedy, note that the word 'natural' does not always mean safe or effective. Scammers add words like 'natural' or 'plant-based' to tempt customers into buying their products. Research the ingredients of any medication you are planning to take and check for allergens or possible drug interactions.

2. Speak to a trusted professional

For all alternative remedies, including vitamins, supplements and other medications, it is imperative that you speak with a trusted healthcare professional before taking them. Your primary care physician or GP will know all of the medications you are on and any treatments you are scheduled to take. Ask them if the treatment you are considering is something they would recommend for you and how it works. Also ask them to run through what the possible side effects are and if it is safe to take as described.

Reminder: if your doctor has never heard of the medication you are being sold, there is probably a reason for that.

3. Improve your online literacy

Finally, be wary of online sites and sellers and brush up on your online literacy and security skills to ensure you are not falling victim to online scammers. Search for courses to help you build up or refresh these skills – places like your local library might offer classes that can help with this. Question everything you see and research products, devices or courses that claim to cure everything.

> ### Reflections
>
> Have you ever fallen victim to a health and well-being scam?
>
> How did it impact your physical, mental and emotional health?

4
Lifestyle

1. Social life   169
2. Leaving the house   175
3. Daily living   183
4. Hospital visits and medical admin   211

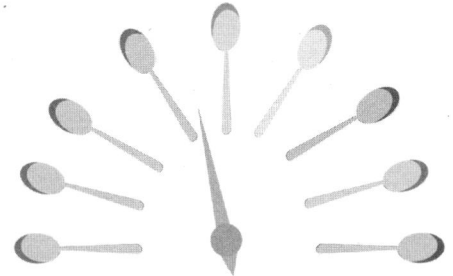

1
Social life

When living with a chronic illness, condition or disability it is easy to feel frustrated and isolated from your loved ones. As spoonies, it can be hard to leave the house on the best of days, let alone during high-symptom days and flare-ups, so when friends and family make plans to go out, spend time together and do new and exciting things, it can be hard to join in. This sense of isolation is especially acute if you have previously been able-bodied and very socially active. Luckily, there are a few things you can do to help yourself, and the people who want to spend time with you, which I will explain below.

Isolation

Personally, I struggle with isolation a lot. When loved ones invite me to events or make plans to do activities together, sometimes the only thought in my head is, 'Sounds like fun. I'll be in pain that day.' When you experience chronic symptoms or disabilities, it can be difficult to look forward to things, knowing you will not have a day off from your condition and that there's a high chance that you'll need to cancel at the last minute.

Even so, it is important to go out, socialise and distract yourself from your pain and symptoms as and when you are able to. If you don't, it is easy for spoonies to wallow in their own misery and become depressed, which can make physical symptoms worse (as discussed on p. 77). For this reason, try to remain at least somewhat socially active, even when it is difficult to do so.

Remaining social also helps to maintain relationships and avoid rejection. People inevitably give up on asking you to things if you continually turn them down or pull out at the last minute, even though your reasons for doing so are totally valid, so it's worth trying to say yes to the important events.

That said, spoonies should also ensure we are resting and pacing ourselves enough to protect our energy and avoid flare-ups. As you can see, getting the balance right between maintaining a social life and preserving our health can be difficult to manage! You will likely sometimes overdo the fun stuff with family and friends and have a flare-up, making you regret joining in.

My tips to avoid social isolation, learned through years of trial and error, are:

- Accept invitations from loved ones when you can
- Ensure you are not overdoing it
- Rest as much as possible before, during and after the event
- Turn down any invitations that you know will lead to flare-ups

Socialise the spoonie way

A great way to socialise more and still be able to manage your own chronic illness, condition or disability is to change the way you are socialising. If going out feels like too much for you, why not try staying in with family and friends instead? Table 7, on the next page, contains some other spoonie-friendly ideas, but you can come up with your own list.

Table 7 Spoonie-friendly socialising

Instead of this...	Try this...
Going to the cinema	Have a movie night at home
Going to a restaurant	Order takeout from the restaurant
Hosting a dinner party	Have guests each bring a dish

These types of easy swaps mean your needs are being looked after and you can avoid overdoing it, while still socialising and having a good time with your loved ones. It is important that you explain to them why these alternatives are beneficial to you, and that they understand why you need to change the way you socialise. This will ensure you are able to accept invitations, while protecting your own physical and mental health needs. It benefits them, too, since you'll be much less likely to cancel, and they'll get to spend time with you when you're at your best, not struggling and in pain and wishing you'd said no.

Community column

'I promise, real friends stick around and try to understand. Just be honest with them and yourself.' – Rachel

'When I have to cancel at the last minute something I've been looking forward to for weeks/months, I am genuinely gutted. People seem to think that I can push through it to do what I want to do, but my body just won't let me. If I say I can't come last minute, just know I tried my hardest and I'm probably crying over the fact I had to cancel.' – Chloe

Loss of relationships

When a spoonie becomes socially isolated it can lead to a loss of the relationships they may have once relied upon. Sadly, the fact is, prioritising your own mental and physical health by declining invitations during high-symptom days or times when you don't have many spare spoons can rub some people up the wrong way.

If someone invites their chronically ill or disabled loved one to multiple different outings or events and keep getting rejected, of course it can be frustrating for them. They may not understand that their spoonie simply cannot join them every time, or even most of the time. This can be perceived as the spoonie purposely choosing to distance themself or simply not putting in enough effort to keep the relationship going. This can be irritating and hurtful, especially if they do not understand why it is happening. And, even if they know you are ill, it can still be a difficult thing to process.

Unfortunately, this kind of disconnect between two parties, where one doesn't understand the circumstances surrounding their loved one's symptoms and feelings and the spoonie themself may be unable to successfully communicate their situation, can lead to a breakdown of the relationship and eventually mean that both parties go their separate ways. This may not be surprising when it occurs, but that does not mean it is not still painful.

My best advice to you is to make sure you and your needs are your priority. Ensure you are doing what is best for your body and your illness because the only one who will suffer the consequences of doing too much is you.

You can also try explaining the situation to the able-bodied person or people (again!). They can likely understand that it's difficult for you to leave the house when you are in pain, but they may not quite comprehend pacing or that you need to conserve your energy and allocate it wisely. A good way to explain this would be to use the spoon theory metaphor, which was designed for exactly this purpose. Tell them how each task will cost a certain number of spoons and that these units of energy are finite and cannot be easily replenished. Having a better understanding of this may help them put things into perspective and be more tolerant and patient.

Ultimately, though, people who cannot understand and empathise with you are not the type of people you need around you. If they decide to cut that relationship off, I view that as a good thing. They should be prioritising themselves and their needs, and you should be doing the same.

> ## Community column
>
> 'Unfortunately, my family isn't a strong system for me because of constant criticism, judgement and gaslighting. My friends, on the other hand, are so accommodating. My friends are truly my strongest support system.' – Becky
>
> 'The toll the pain takes on romantic relationships [is great]: living with a partner in chronic pain is not for the faint of heart or people who need constant uplifting. Because unfortunately living in chronic pain leaves us with more "bad" days than good.' – Jennifer

Now, I'd like to speak to those loved ones we sometimes need to cancel on: this bit is for you.

I know how annoying it is to be cancelled on at the very last minute, especially when it happens more than once. I empathise; I really do. I also hate last-minute changes and when people cancel. However, it is important that you remember that as frustrating as our illness may be to you, it is infinitely more frustrating for us. We have to live in a body that is malfunctioning, that simply will not co-operate. A body that we cannot predict or control and that is failing us. The person you know and love would dearly like to be 'normal', but we are not. We are not able to do all of the things we want to, or all of the things you may want us to do. It is perfectly natural for you to get frustrated with us when we cancel at the last minute, but please remember to show some compassion, too.

> **Reflections**
>
> Have you experienced a loss of relationships due to your chronic illness?
>
> What would you say to that person today?

2
Leaving the house

When you have a disability or chronic illness it can be difficult to plan a fun day out, but it is definitely still possible with a little extra forethought. The point of this chapter is to highlight some of the things that we spoonies need to focus on when we make plans to leave the house and socialise.

> Please note that some of the factors discussed in this chapter are issues that able-bodied people may also need to consider, such as financial planning and outfit choices. This chapter is not meant to belittle the needs of able-bodied people, but to highlight the special needs of spoonies.

Planning ahead

Although able-bodied people also need to plan days out, it is undoubtedly much more difficult for a spoonie and will likely take us much longer. This is simply because there are many additional factors we need to take into consideration and more planning and forethought is required for us to be safe and comfortable. We cannot 'go with the flow' and 'see what happens', which makes it difficult to be spontaneous and impulsive.

To help things run smoothly, here is a list of factors that you might want to consider before you leave your home:

1. Accessibility
2. Tickets
3. Finances
4. Travel
5. Rest
6. Medications
7. Mobility aids
8. Outfit
9. Food and drink

1. Accessibility

Before deciding on a place to visit, it is important that you ensure the venue is accessible and suited to your needs. This can mean it has step-free or wheelchair access, space to manoeuvre with mobility aids, a disabled toilet, high-contrast signage and hearing loop functions, or anything else you may require during your visit. An individual's access needs can differ from day to day, and it is imperative that all of these are fulfilled correctly so that we can enjoy ourselves when out and about. Nowadays this information is usually listed online, though unfortunately sometimes the full details are not available or up to date, so it can take time to determine whether the venue is suitable. Also, many venues that claim to be accessible are not in fact so, which can lead to disappointment on the day.

So, do plenty of research beforehand. Call the venue, especially if your needs are more complex. You can also read reviews and social media posts about the venue, to gain a better understanding of its accessibility.

2. Tickets

Some venues may require disabled people to purchase specific tickets, so they are aware of your disability and can keep a count of exactly how many disabled people will be at the venue at a specific time and date. This is usually seen at places such as theatres or cinemas where there's a limited number of wheelchair and step-free accessible seats for disabled people.

Furthermore, some places will offer disabled people tickets at a concession price. This makes the ticket slightly cheaper and thus more affordable. This usually needs to be pre-booked with evidence of a disability, such as a disabled parking permit or a letter from your doctor. In addition, some venues also offer a free carer ticket with proof of disability. All of this requires extra research when planning days out and many need to be booked in advance.

3. Finances

More expensive plans take more forward planning. Often, disabled people are unable to work at all, or at least significantly fewer hours than their able-bodied peers (*see* p. 137 for more on this). This can mean their disposable income is much smaller than that of those around them. Personally, I am unable to work and so I am usually not able to spend much money on fun outings and going to exciting new places. This can be a difficult factor to discuss, especially with family and friends who may then offer to pay for your share of an outing. I prefer to pay my own way and do not like to accept money from people, especially when I know I would struggle to pay them back.

All of this means that spontaneous plans and last-minute outings can be difficult to commit to when you are a spoonie. Bigger outings and more expensive events will usually require a decent notice period so a spoonie has enough time to save and plan ahead.

4. Travel

Forward planning when it comes to travel arrangements for disabled and chronically ill people is an absolute must. Whether you plan to drive or use public transport, there are several things you need to know:

By car If you plan to drive to a venue, it is imperative that you know where the nearest parking spaces are, whether or not disabled parking is available and exactly how close it is to the venue. If the walking distance from your car to the venue is too far, it will be difficult for you to have enough energy to complete it. Prior research is always a necessity for this and sometimes we will need to purchase a parking space ahead of time to ensure we can park close to the venue.

By public transport If you decide to take public transport you may need to know how to get through the journey with step-free access, wheelchair assistance, hearing loop functions or with a service animal. This requires planning and forethought to ensure that the journey is accessible to us, and that our accommodations are taken into account.

It is also important to respect your own limitations and assess your available spoons when using public transport. A journey that takes over an hour, for example, can be exhausting, both physically and mentally. If you need to travel for that long, you should consider whether you'll then have the available spoons to do your activity, before making another journey home again.

By taxi Planning a journey in a taxi has its own challenges. We may need to book a cab that allows service animals, has a ramp for a wheelchair or space in the back for our mobility aids to be safely stored. This can add to the cost of the taxi ride. It can also be difficult to find a cab that has everything we need plus a driver who is at least somewhat knowledgeable in how to handle our mobility aids. The high cost and these extra requirements can mean that 'just booking a cab' is not a viable option for us, so booking ahead is vital.

5. Rest

Planning a day out requires plenty of rest both before and after the event (*see* pacing, p. 64). Most able-bodied people can do a different activity every day without needing time off in between, but most spoonies simply cannot do that.

Personally, I try to schedule my own plans to ensure I have at least two rest days before a big event and one or two days afterwards, too. I have found this to be the most beneficial to me. If you have a more strenuous activity planned, you may need to rest for longer afterwards, whereas if you have a less exhausting plan you may not need that long to rest beforehand.

In my opinion, it is better to get more rest than less, so I always overestimate how much rest I will need. However, I also know that I am privileged to be able to do that and it simply isn't always an option for people with work and children or other commitments. Whatever your situation, try to find the right balance that works for you and make sure you are not overscheduling and overexerting yourself.

6. Medications

When planning trips, whether for just a day out or longer, pre-planning to ensure you have enough medication on hand is a must. This includes your regularly scheduled medication but might also cover some extra painkillers and other medicines in case you experience additional symptoms while out and about.

Advance notice may also be needed to ensure you can stop any medicine that has side effects you may not want to deal with outside the home. For example, if a particular medication causes vomiting or diarrhoea, you may decide to skip a dose (if it is safe to do so) to avoid these additional symptoms on the day out.

When travelling abroad, please check local laws and airline rules about prescription medications, since some countries have very strict laws about narcotics, for instance. You should also ensure that you have appropriate travel insurance that covers you for emergency care and/or prescriptions if you need it.

7. Mobility aids

The mobility aids that spoonies may need can change due to a number of different factors, including many things that are outside of our control. These include sleep, medications, current symptom levels, location and projected symptom levels. Having the time, energy and space to bring our mobility aids with us can take extra planning. For example, if an ambulatory wheelchair user needs their wheelchair on a day out, they will need to ensure that their access needs are met with step-free travel arrangements, a step-free venue and space to manoeuvre, etc. If plans were made assuming that person would not need their wheelchair, those plans must then be re-examined to ensure they are still suitable for a wheelchair user.

8. Outfit

Like most people, we spoonies will need to plan an outfit that is suitable for the venue we are going to be visiting. However, unlike most people, we may need to decide on an outfit based on our symptoms. For example, we might need to avoid tight clothes if our pain level is high, or buckles and buttons if arthritis is flaring up, or certain textures due to skin irritations or sensory issues. In addition, it may be necessary to pack extra clothes to bring with us in case of other issues, like spills due to tremors or accidents due to incontinence. These things all need forward planning and extra thought.

9. Food and drink

Often, we will need to research the food and drink that may be available during an outing. Some medications have to be taken with food, in which case it is impossible for us to simply skip a meal or wait until we get home. Therefore, it is important that we know what the available food options are as well as the cost of a meal or snack, as affording it may require further budgeting. We may also need to know if there are any alternative options for people with allergies or intolerances.

Furthermore, it is necessary to know whether a venue will allow us to bring in outside food in case the food options available are not suitable. If a venue does not allow this, it can be a dealbreaker.

> **Reflections**
>
> Do you routinely plan adequate rest days before and after a day out?
>
> Are there any other factors you need to consider when planning to socialise outside the home?

3

Daily living

Chronic illness and disability will touch virtually every part of your life, and as much as you might wish it otherwise, your life will not look the same as it once did. The good news is that by being adaptable and learning to roll with the punches, you will be able to acclimatise to your new reality and find ways of carrying on. Your schedule will look different, the way you carry out basic tasks like cooking and cleaning will look different and the way you run errands will look different, but that's OK. You just need to find techniques to make your new normal work for you.

In this chapter I'll be sharing some top tips and hacks for surviving day to day when you live with a chronic illness, condition or disability, because running a household is something that a lot of spoonies struggle with. I know I certainly do! The routine of cooking and cleaning can be difficult when there is absolutely nothing routine about our bodies and the symptoms we experience on a daily basis.

Cleaning your home

Keeping a clean and well-maintained home is vital for your physical and mental health. A sanitary and tidy home environment gives us a safe space to rest and recover in peace and stops us from becoming overwhelmed by sensory input that can contribute to poor mental health. However, it can be difficult to maintain and clean our living spaces when we have an illness or disability to also deal with. How can I chip away at the mountain of laundry piling up when I can't even guarantee I'll be able to get out of bed in the morning?

So what's my number one tip to make sure your house is perfectly clean and tidy all year round? Answer: give up on this dream now.

Your house is probably never going to be a flawlessly neat, impeccably tidy, Instagram-able haven. Setting the bar that high will inevitably lead to disappointment. If you can't afford a team of cleaners to come in every day then your house is unlikely to be perfectly spotless all the time. But don't despair: it can still be clean, and I can show you how!

So, here are my best tips for staying on top of the household cleaning:

1. Stay organised
2. Prioritise visible mess
3. Adapt the task
4. Prioritise your list
5. Ask for help
6. Know your limitations

1. Stay organised

First, in order to keep on top of your housework you should try to stay organised. Make a list and check it twice – just like Santa Claus. Create a daily list of things you *need* to do and whittle it down to the things you *can* do. Bear in mind that overexerting yourself will only cause problems and is not a good idea. The key is consistency to ensure you are managing your to-do list on a regular basis.

In terms of staying organised, I find lists are the most helpful to me to keep on track. For this reason I have created a cleaning schedule that I try my best to use myself. This allows me to clearly see what tasks need to happen within my home and how often they need to be carried out. Take the example in table 8, below, and make it your own so that it works for you, your family and your household.

Table 8 Example cleaning schedule

Daily	Weekly	Monthly	Seasonally	Yearly
Make the bed	Mop floors	Clean kitchen door fronts	Wash pillows and duvets	Deep-clean carpets
Wash the dishes	Dust	Clean light switches and door handles	Clean skirting boards	Clean fireplaces
Load and unload the dishwasher	Clean bathrooms	Clean oven and microwave	Wash throws and blankets	Organise storage areas
Clean countertops	Change dustbin bags	Clean the dishwasher	Sort/clear out wardrobes	Purge clutter
Clean the sink	Clean the stove	Clean the windows	Organise kitchen cabinets	Check light bulbs
Do the laundry	Clear the fridge of any expired food	Clean mirrors	Clean and organise the freezer	
General pick-up	Hoover stairs and bedrooms			
Sweep floors				
Take out rubbish and recycling				

This cleaning template is one I created to help me remember what needs to be done, when and how frequently. It is important to remember that everyone's ideal cleaning schedule will look different dependent on your own needs and standards. In a perfect world I'd have no issue sticking to this schedule but in reality, it can be very difficult to manage daily tasks, and the larger tasks, though infrequent, can be hard to do alone. Even though I created this schedule, I struggle to carry out the tasks on it fully, and honestly, there's no shame in that. I do the best that I can at any given time and I'm not ashamed of that fact. And neither should you be.

2. Prioritise visible mess

I have found that it is essential to focus on the most visible mess first. This is because by cleaning up and tidying the most on-show and high-traffic areas, you will be able to cut down on the sensory overload that mess can cause. If you run out of spoons immediately afterwards, you can at least rest knowing you've tackled the most important parts already.

So, ask yourself what your top-priority areas are. What is the most visible and highly noticeable mess and what needs to be done to make it look cleaner and tidier? This is probably going to be different for every household and it will usually depend on your own and your family's needs.

In my home the most visible mess is found in the kitchen area and the living room. This is where everyone spends most of their time, including visitors. I therefore like these spaces to be fairly clean and tidy so as not to be totally embarrassing. Figure out what areas you need to prioritise within your home and start by tackling those places first.

3. Adapt the task

My next piece of advice is to adapt the task to yourself. As someone with multiple chronic illnesses and chronic pain, my mobility can be limited. I have a hard time bending and stretching as well as sitting and standing for long periods. Therefore, in order for me to do daily cleaning tasks around my house I need to adapt them to suit my body and the symptoms I'm experiencing at the time.

Home aids, gadgets and various cleaning hacks can be a lifesaver when it comes to adapting tasks. I have several that I use to help me carry out chores and save some time and energy. Let's explore some of these now:

Recycling/general waste bins Separated bins for recycling and general waste make it much easier to recycle the correct materials. If these bins are large-capacity, you should need to change them less often. On the flip side, rubbish bins that are too big will have heavier bags and this can make it harder to carry rubbish outside. Find the right method for you or get help with taking heavy rubbish and recycling sacks out.

Long-handled pan and brush I use my long-handled dustpan and brush set so that I never need to bend to pick up piles of rubbish. The lightweight design makes it easier to use than a regular-sized, heavy broom, which means I am much more likely to stay on top of the task even when I'm experiencing symptoms like pain and fatigue. In our house, we've found it a good idea to keep one set upstairs and one downstairs, for easier access.

Lightweight broom and mop As well as a long-handled pan and brush, a lightweight regular broom and mop are essentials. If your cleaning items are too heavy, they will be of very little use to you, as you'll need more energy to use them. If your items are lightweight but durable, you can clean even when you have symptoms.

Hand-held hoover A hand-held hoover is good for cleaning hard-to-reach areas, upholstered furniture and pet areas without needing to get the heavy full-sized hoover out. Hand-held hoovers are also cheaper, easier to maintain and will likely get more use than a full-sized hoover. Personally, I have found it beneficial to invest a bit more money in a good-quality one, for the long battery life and strong suction.

Long-handled grabber Avoid bending by using a long-handled grabber to pick up medium to large items from the floor or other hard-to-reach areas in your home. These grabbers are usually made of lightweight materials and are relatively cheap, making them widely accessible. The drawback is that it can be difficult to pick up smaller or quite heavy items and using them takes a little practice.

No-bend laundry basket A raised laundry basket is great for getting your laundry done without needing to bend too much. Many will come with wheels, so they can be dragged with ease. Wheeled baskets will also usually have brakes on them, and some come with extra storage space for pegs or other small items, making them handy for use indoors or outdoors. They can sometimes be a little more expensive than the regular ones, but if you are the one responsible for laundry in your home, the investment may be worth it.

Long-handled scrub brush These are good for cleaning hard-to-reach areas like skirting boards and in bathrooms for areas such as the bathtub, tiles, the shower tray and the floor without needing to bend too much or causing too much fatigue. Electric or automatic scrubbers are also available, and they need less elbow grease and get things cleaner faster. Unfortunately, electric scrubbers can get quite pricey so they are more of an investment; do some research to find out what will work best for you.

4. Prioritise your list

You're also going to need to prioritise your to-do list. It's all well and good putting ten things on your list but if your body physically cannot do all those tasks, what's the point? If you're anything like me it will just frustrate you that you can't do them all, even though you already know if you push yourself too far, you'll have a flare-up and regret it later when you can't make it across the room to get a snack.

In fact, prioritising your tasks is such an important point that we're going to take a closer look at it now.

Prioritising your to-do list

In this section I will run through an example of a to-do list and how I would go about handling it. Remember, my opinions on what is important and necessary may be different to yours, so make it your own and personalise the techniques I have outlined as much as you need to.

Kitchen jobs

- Clean and put away the dishes
- Clean the countertops
- Sweep the floor
- Mop the floor
- Organise the pantry
- Sort and clean the fridge and freezer
- Clean the microwave
- Clean the stovetop
- Clean the oven

This is a fairly average list of jobs for the daily, weekly or monthly maintenance of most kitchens, and for many able-bodied people it probably wouldn't be that difficult to do all of these things over a few sessions, or even in a single go if they have a lot of time and energy. However, for us spoonies, completing these tasks will be more difficult. Our bodies are different, our needs are different, and our priorities are different.

So, let's make a few adjustments to this list to make it a bit more manageable for us. First, we'll decide how much of a priority the job is. If it's a high priority it stays on the list; if it's a low priority it can wait until we have more available spoons. We'll also decide if there is an adaptation we can make to help us complete the task and save some spoons. Don't forget that whether a task is a high priority or not depends on your needs, your home and your family's situation. So what I've listed in table 9, on the next page, is just a reflection of my own opinions.

Table 9 Kitchen jobs

Task	Priority	Adaptation
Clean and put away the dishes	High	Sit down
Clean the countertops	High	None
Sweep the floor	Medium	Long dustpan/brush
Mop the floor	Low	None
Organise the pantry	Low	Sit down
Sort and clean the fridge and freezer	Medium	Sit down
Clean the microwave	Medium	None
Clean the stovetop	Medium	Sit down
Clean the oven	Low	Self-clean function

Therefore, taking these points into consideration, my new to-do list would look something like this:

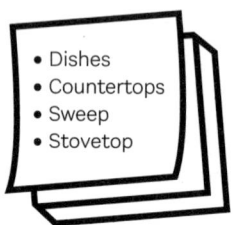

- Dishes
- Countertops
- Sweep
- Stovetop

These four jobs have been kept on the list because they are all either one or more of these:

- Highly visible, so completing them will instantly make the overall appearance of the kitchen much better (e.g. cleaning the countertops and stovetop)
- Adjustable, so I can change the way I do them to suit my needs by adding a chair or other aid to help me complete the task (e.g. sweeping the floor with a long-handled brush)
- A priority, so due to my and my family's needs these jobs are the most urgent that need to be completed (e.g. cleaning and putting away the dishes)

Breaking down my to-do lists in this way has allowed me to successfully keep on top of the regular chores that need to be done on a daily or weekly basis. When it comes to tasks that are carried out more infrequently, such as monthly or seasonal tasks, I try to reserve them for days when I have much more time and energy and far fewer overall symptoms. This means that my home looks tidy and clean but that I am not overdoing it and pushing myself past my natural limitations.

5. Ask for help

This tip is one of the most important. Ask for help! If others live in your household they can do a lot of the heavy lifting and more difficult tasks, as well as their fair share of the day-to-day tasks. For example, I struggle to lift heavy items and cannot easily bend. Therefore, I will ask someone else in my house to carry the basket of clean laundry back upstairs.

It can be difficult to ask for help, but a huge lesson I've learned throughout my chronic illness journey is that I physically cannot do it alone and trying to do so will lead to nothing but flare-ups and frustration. I need the people around me, and accepting their help is not a weakness or a personal failing. This is something I wish I had realised much earlier, as it could have saved me a lot of spoons and pain, but that's why I'm sharing it with you now.

6. Know your limitations

Another big lesson that I have learned is how to manage my own expectations of myself. It has taken me a very long time to understand my own abilities and limitations and the fact that they regularly fluctuate has made that even more challenging. It takes a lot of self-reflection and patience to view yourself clearly in the way that's necessary when you live with a chronic illness, condition or disability. You need to understand and constantly assess your body.

Reminder: if you take just one thing from this book, I want it to be this: take the time to learn about yourself, your needs, your priorities and your limitations. It is the best way to manage your spoonie life on a daily basis, and in the wider scope of things, too.

This also applies when it comes to keeping your house clean. Remember your own limitations and restrictions. Having a clean home is important, but so is your physical and mental health and well-being. Pushing yourself too far is simply not worth the consequences it brings at the end of the day. Remember the steps we discussed about prioritising your to-do list and adapting tasks to ensure they are not costing too many spoons to carry out.

> **Reflections**
>
> How do you currently tackle household chores like cleaning?
>
> What is one tip from this chapter that you could implement in your own life?

Preparing and cooking meals

Preparing and cooking meals when you have a chronic illness, condition or disability can be very difficult. The physical task can be tough, as pain and symptoms can mean we don't always have the energy or ability to do it. Symptoms and side effects such as low appetite and nausea can also add to the difficulty of the task, as well as the fact that it's also quite a mentally draining process.

In our home, I am often responsible for cooking dinner every night and I have personally felt this burden very intensely in the past. In order to relieve this strain I've come up with some ways to make things easier at every stage of the process by breaking up the meal planning and cooking process into smaller steps:

1. Planning
2. Organising

3. Prepping
4. Cooking

1. Planning

A little planning can go a long way towards making life easier, so try to develop a few habits that work for you. These are mine:

- Keep a running list of what is in your fridge, freezer and pantry, especially any meat products, cooked items or short-shelf-life items
- Use a weekly menu planner to decide what meals to serve and when. Place it in a visible area, such as on the fridge door, so your family will stop asking you what's for dinner every five minutes (yeah, right!)
- Make a list of meals you know you and your family like to eat so you can just pick a few during the planning stage
- Be prepared to scrap your plans if you are unable to cook that day, due to symptom flare-ups or lack of energy

2. Organising

Online shopping is of course one simple option (see p. 197), but if you do decide you want to go to the shops in person, the following apply:

- Go grocery shopping with a list of everything you need for the week's meals, so you don't forget anything and need to go out again
- Group your shopping list by section to avoid going around the store multiple times (e.g. group fridge items together, frozen items together, etc.)
- Go grocery shopping with another person if you can, so they can pick up the slack if you are not feeling well
- Shop on a day when you have sufficient spoons and try to avoid peak times where there are more people around and the queues will be much longer

3. Prepping

It's all very well planning and buying your food, but now you need to prepare it. These top tips help reduce the strain for me:

- Defrost meat and other items overnight in the fridge. Leave yourself a note or set a reminder so you don't forget to do this
- Use pre-cut fruits and vegetables if possible or cut them in advance so you are not prepping and cooking at the same time
- Get all of your ingredients, utensils and cookware out at once so you don't forget things you need or have to go back and forth, wasting valuable spoons
- Have a copy of your recipe to hand, to help you keep track of things. Save it on your phone or print a copy if you need to

4. Cooking

Once everything is prepped, you can move on to the cooking stage, either immediately or after a rest. These hacks will hopefully make it all a bit easier:

- Cook meals sitting down if you can: using a stool or chair by the stove works wonders
- Use tools, gadgets and home aids to assist you when cooking (see below for more)
- Cook the majority of the meal earlier in the day and finish it off in the evening if it helps conserve your spoons. For example, prep, cook and layer your lasagne in the afternoon and bake it in the evening
- Batch-cook larger quantities and freeze leftovers in regular portion sizes for a quick meal another time

Aids that can help with cooking and eating

I have found various aids, gadgets and equipment that help me with the tasks in the kitchen that I struggle with. My favourites are listed below.

Tall chair/perching stool

Perfect for use during cooking and cleaning tasks, a lightweight, easily moveable chair or stool can be a great addition to your kitchen. I use mine for prepping food, cooking at the stove, washing dishes and cleaning and organising cupboards and drawers.

Slow cooker

This is great for days when you have limited energy or lots of symptoms, since you just throw your ingredients in and let the cooker do the hard work. It's an excellent option in winter for stews and soups. Research cookers with a good energy rating to ensure the cost of running it does not outweigh the benefits of using it.

Microwave

A lifesaver in the kitchen, a microwave is excellent for reheating leftovers, quickly defrosting the food you forgot to get out of the freezer last night and, in a pinch, cooking instant foods like ready meals when you simply have no spoons left.

Cups and bowls with lids

Cups and bowls with lids are excellent for transferring food and drink from place to place with very little spillage, especially if you have tremors. If you have issues with hand strength and mobility, dishes with handles are an excellent option, too. Another good idea is using lightweight plastic dishes so that your items are not too heavy to use. Children's dishes or picnicware are affordable, easily accessible options.

Rotary or automatic cheese grater

Rotary graters are excellent if you have the hand and arm strength to use the rotating function, but an electric grater is a good alternative if you'd prefer the auto feature. Either is great for grating and slicing cheese as well as fruits, vegetables and other various ingredients.

Automatic can opener

These are fantastic for opening canned goods with very little effort and will help you access easy meals with very little prep (beans on toast, anyone?).

Jar and bottle opener

A specific jar and bottle opener is a great aid to keep on hand, as it can make food and drink easier to access and prepare. In fact, it is useful for anyone regardless of whether they have a chronic illness or not!

Lap tray or folding side table

Both are very good options for eating on the sofa or in bed without worrying about spills and crumbs. They are also great for working or relaxing on the sofa or in bed during high-symptom days and flare-ups.

Ergonomic cutlery

Some cutlery is made specifically for people with arm and hand weakness or mobility issues and is designed with people who have arthritis in mind. These items can take the pressure off your fingers, hands and wrists and help you in the long run.

Reminder: there is no shame in needing extra assistance. Just because others wouldn't need additional aid to get the job done, it does not mean you shouldn't use one if you need one.

> ### Reflections
>
> How do you handle cooking and eating tasks on a daily basis?
>
> What is one tip from this chapter that you could implement in your own life?

Running errands

Running errands when you have a chronic illness, condition or disability can be difficult; we face so many more challenges than the able-bodied people around us that even something as basic as going to the post office might become a nightmare. Experience has taught me a lot and so here are some words of wisdom that might save you from some of the many, many mistakes I've made over the years.

Grocery shopping

Nowadays it is very common for major supermarkets to offer online shopping options and delivery services, and using these is one of the best ways to save your precious spoons. You can have groceries delivered to your door, at the time and date of your choosing, with very little fuss (and barely any social interaction). This saves you struggling to go out, select items, bag them up, carry them and deal with bringing them in. Delivery slots will often vary in cost based on time and day, but if you are available, off-peak times are usually much cheaper and have more availability.

There is a negative aspect to online grocery shopping, though. Personally, when I go shopping, I like to feel the fruits and vegetables to find the best stuff and I check the back of the shelf to get the freshest items, with the longest use-by dates. Yep, I'm one of *those* people. Employees who pick your items for you for online delivery may not always select the freshest produce or items with a long use-by date, so the groceries that you receive may not be up to your standards. If that is something that is important to you, bear that in mind when you are doing your online shop.

Anyone who has done an online grocery shop will know all about substitutions. When an item is out of stock, no longer in store or unavailable, a similar item is chosen as a substitute, unless you tick a box saying you do not want this, in which case you will get nothing. If you need a specific brand or quantity, then both the substitute and the no-item option can become an issue, especially if you have allergies or food intolerances or want to make a specific dish. To solve the problem, you can usually choose a specific item that pickers can substitute if your preferred item is unavailable.

For some people, the added cost of home delivery is an issue that stops them from online shopping. Delivery slots can be quite pricey, especially at peak and busy times such as over Christmas or school holidays. To offset this, some supermarkets offer click and collect services. This means you order your items online in the same way, they are picked and packed in store, and then you drive to the pick-up zone to collect your shopping. This service is sometimes free, but when there is a charge, it is usually cheaper than an at-home delivery service. This cuts out walking around the shop but means you will still have to unload your shopping and bring it inside your home yourself.

Overall, when it comes to online grocery shopping there are plenty of options; it is just a matter of finding out what works for you. Don't forget, our conditions can change and fluctuate quite regularly. If one week you feel well enough to shop in person, that's great news. But online shopping is a good fallback for when your symptoms are flaring up and you simply cannot handle walking around a shop, bending to find items and carrying them back.

Prescriptions

When it comes to obtaining prescription medications, things can get a bit overwhelming. If you're like me, you may be on several different medications and they probably all come in at different times, so you might find yourself in and out of the pharmacy and seeing the pharmacist behind the counter more often than you see your friends. If this is you, don't worry, I've got some tips for managing the situation.

Collection

For some people, manually collecting your prescriptions makes the most sense. You can speak to your pharmacist and get advice, ask questions and be served by an actual human being. Plus, if you're out and about anyway, why not just stop off quickly and grab what you need? It makes sense. Some people with chronic illnesses even use collecting their prescription as a way to get out of the house. For years, I did this myself. After university, I was unable to work and so I found myself home alone most days. Having a reason to go out and something to do helped not only my mental health but walking the very short distance to the pharmacy was a nice way to get some gentle (and free) exercise.

So, for all of these reasons, collecting your prescriptions in person can be a good idea. My advice if you do this is to try to group orders of your medications together so that they will need refilling at the same time, so you don't have to go out every other day to get different items. Sometimes syncing all of your repeat prescriptions might take some co-ordination with the prescribing doctor (or possibly their secretary) but usually a quick phone call or email will do the trick.

Another piece of advice is calling the pharmacy ahead of time. I hate that thing that happens sometimes when they say, 'Oh, this will be ready on Monday,' so you go out bright and early on Monday morning and when you get there they say, 'Come back in the afternoon; it's not ready yet.' Great. I physically cannot make this journey again today. Now I'll have to wait until tomorrow to come back (if I'm lucky), and I don't have an essential medication I need. Save yourself the headache and call the pharmacy before leaving the house to ask them if your medication is ready and if it is, tell them you are coming to collect it now. That way, they can (hopefully) get it ready to collect and you won't need to wait around too long.

Delivery services

If going in person to collect your prescriptions isn't something you can do, or want to do, prescription delivery services are becoming more and more common nowadays. I personally use one that delivers my medications to my door within a few days of requesting them from my GP, and it's fantastic.

This service is a good fit for me because I experience unpredictable symptoms, which can fluctuate wildly and very quickly, plus flare-ups that can occur for seemingly no reason, or outside factors such as weather. This can make it hard for me to walk to the pharmacy and, as I don't drive, my only other option would be the bus, which can use up a lot of time and spoons. So, switching to a prescription delivery service was the best choice for me.

Most of these types of services will require you to contact your GP directly and have them send your prescriptions to them as usual and, if there are no issues, within a few days they will deliver the medications to your doorstep in discrete packages. As I'm on medications that need to be refrigerated, those are sent in a cool bag, so they remain as cold as possible while in transit. In the past I have had no real issues with the service that I use and would highly recommend it for anyone living with a chronic illness.

Instead of switching to an online pharmacy, you could check with your local pharmacy to see if they offer a delivery service themselves, as this can save time. If your pharmacy does not offer this service, contact your GP or primary care provider to see if they can recommend the name of a trusted online service that they already work with.

Non-grocery shopping

When shopping for clothes and other items I try to do most of my shopping online. This means I can avoid long walks, heavy lifting and waiting in line (as well as other people!). However, sometimes in-person shopping is unavoidable, so here are a few ways I try to make it as easy as possible:

1. Keep a running list
2. Group items
3. Anticipate your needs

1. Keep a running list

I like to keep a running list on my phone, so as soon as I think of something I might need I can jot it down and remember it when I'm out and about. I try to break my list into categories either by item type (clothing, personal items, hobbies, etc.) or by shop. Find a system that works for you, because if you're anything like me you'll be standing in the shop and have forgotten what you came in for.

2. Group items

Instead of going to the shops as soon as I need a single item, I try to wait until I need a few things, so I can get everything at once. I find shopping in person quite exhausting, so by grouping items together and waiting as long as I can manage to, I feel I get more accomplished on my shopping trips. I also try to go on a day where I am experiencing very few symptoms, and in the morning, when I have the most spoons and time.

3. Anticipate your needs

In a similar vein, I find it important to anticipate my own needs. In order to do this, I try to think ahead to the coming weeks and months and see if I can get an early start on shopping. If I'm already planning a shopping trip and know it's a friend's birthday next month, I'll think of a gift and try to figure out if there's anything else I could buy while I'm out buying the present. While I'm there, if I know that I have other friends and family members' birthdays coming up too, I'll just get them all at once. Even if that means I'm weeks and months ahead, I'll just keep the gifts and cards safe at home and add a note in my calendar on that person's birthday notation reminding me that their card is in the bottom drawer of my dresser.

Post office

As someone who enjoys a bit of online shopping (way too much, in fact!) I find myself needing to return and send parcels fairly often. In order to speed this process along a bit I usually purchase and print the labels I need at home so I can avoid long waiting times and sometimes even skip the lines altogether if there is a self-help desk.

Wherever possible, I opt for a collection service to come and pick up my parcels from my home instead of me needing to go myself. This is sometimes offered for free but sometimes requires a small payment. If the item is particularly large, heavy or bulky then I am usually willing to pay the fee, as it's not too expensive and it will save me time and spoons.

Another way I make this whole process easier is by batching parcels together, so I send and return items in groups instead of one at a time. For example, if I have one parcel to send and I am expecting another one soon, I will usually wait as long as I can just in case I need to return the second one, too. In order to do this, it is very important that you know exactly how long you have to return an item. Most of the time it will be one month from the delivery date, but sometimes it is more or less. Do your research to make sure you return items in time.

Finally, when I take packages to the post office or other drop-off points, I will try to get a ride (thanks, Dad!) or I will use my rollator (a mobility aid for stability with a seat and wheels – *see* p. 207). This has a place to put my packages and means I don't have to carry anything too heavy or bulky in my arms. Even lightweight parcels can cause fatigue, pain and other symptoms and overall it is always better to do less lifting and carrying of items wherever possible, by using mobility aids or asking for help from loved ones or carers.

> **Reflections**
>
> What are your top tips for running errands?
>
> What is one tip from this chapter that you could implement in your own life?

Mobility aids

I've mentioned mobility aids a few times throughout this section on lifestyle and elsewhere, whether it's for carrying packages to the post office or helping you access days out, but what actually are they, and who are they for? Let's find out.

Who could benefit from mobility aids?

Something I wish I had understood earlier is that mobility aids are designed to help people with mobility issues enjoy more freedom and independence in their daily lives. The most common mobility aids are:

- Wheelchairs
- Crutches
- Walking sticks/canes
- Rollators
- Walkers/walking frames
- Mobility scooters

Many people think that mobility aids are only for older people, or people who are paralysed and cannot walk. This is simply not true. Mobility aids are for anybody who needs them. Yet making the decision to begin using them can be difficult and deeply personal. Many spoonies struggle because of fear of judgement from others or a belief that they are 'not disabled enough' to need one. This misplaced view can hold people back from using something that will genuinely make their life better.

However, if you are even half thinking about getting a mobility aid, you probably already need one. People who don't need a mobility aid don't sit around debating if they should get one, so the fact that you're even considering it means that you likely need it.

My own decision to begin using mobility aids was tricky. As a young disabled woman I did not want to draw attention to the fact that my health was in decline. I feared what people, including friends and family, would think of me when they saw the aids. As a result of this, I suffered for much longer than I should have; I pretended I wasn't getting worse as days went by and as well as my physical health declining, my mental health did too. At the time I did not understand that using a mobility aid would set me free, give me confidence and independence, and that it wasn't a sign that I had 'given up'.

Community column

'It was hard for me to accept I needed some form of support to walk with during my flare-ups. Being a mum of energetic young boys I need to get around but felt I didn't want to look like I had a disability. So I opted for crutches. It's made such a difference when we are out.' – Jenni

It is essential that anybody who may require a mobility aid(s) uses one, because ignoring your needs can cause greater harm and possibly even long-term damage. The idea that you are 'letting yourself down' simply by using the mobility aids your body requires is ableist and harmful. Never let anybody tell you these things. If they do, they are wrong.

Mobility aids can:

- Reduce your chances of falling over
- Improve confidence and self-esteem
- Reduce joint pain and pressure
- Give you better balance
- Provide a place to sit when you need to rest
- Provide a storage space so you don't need to carry things
- Give you independence and freedom
- Help you walk longer distances
- Reduce pain
- Increase stability

Reminder: never be ashamed of knowing what your body needs, understanding your limitations and adjusting your life accordingly. It is so important to live your life according to who you actually are, and not who people think you are.

Which mobility aid is right for me?

In this section we will discuss how to go about figuring out which mobility aid may suit your needs. There are several questions you can ask yourself to assess which will work for you, and answering honestly is an important step to figuring this out. To begin, you need to understand yourself and your needs. Ask yourself:

- How often do you require a mobility aid? Every day? Some days? Just during flare-ups?

This will help you to understand whether you require a daily aid or something tailored to your flare-up symptoms.

- Are you physically independent? Can you perform daily tasks without assistance? Can you walk outdoors?

If the answer to these questions is no, you may require a wheelchair or mobility scooter.

- Do you need two-handed supports?

If you have more balance issues, a two-sided support can be a great help, from something such as a rollator or walker.

- Do you need single-sided support?

If you need single-sided support, a cane or walking stick might be better suited to you. There are several types on the market, including a seated cane (if you tire easily), a quad cane (for greater stability) and a single-point cane. Try a few options and see what works best for you.

Other things you may need to consider are the overall costs of the mobility aids, including the outright cost of purchasing one and any maintenance and upkeep they may require (such as for wheelchairs and mobility scooters). Unfortunately, some mobility aids may be prohibitively expensive and you may require a cheaper alternative or help with funding. In cases where money is an issue there may be charity or government schemes that can help you buy the aids you require and even schemes to help alter your home to your needs. It is important that you use official sources such as government websites or charity helplines to find information about these grants and schemes.

Personally, I use a rollator when I walk longer distances or need to carry items (such as when I am shopping), two crutches at home when I need support on both sides but cannot manoeuvre my rollator in the narrow spaces, or a walking stick for single-sided support and for walking short distances. Needing multiple mobility aids for different scenarios is not out of the ordinary and you may find having a range useful for your situation, too.

Regardless of the type of mobility aid that you require it is important to get one that works best for your needs. If you need a wheelchair, there are many options, such as manual, motorised, self-propelled or a pushchair that requires a caregiver. Do plenty of research before choosing, and ensure you are purchasing from a reputable seller. Before committing to a wheelchair, which can be expensive, look into rental options so you can try one out before you buy.

When deciding between walking sticks and canes, take into consideration the type you may need, the length and the handle. If you wear different shoes for different occasions it may be best to get a height-adjustable stick rather than a fixed-height stick. This will ensure that regardless of the height of your shoes, you are getting the correctly adjusted height of stick, and it is correctly positioned to give you maximum support. Also take into consideration the type of handle your stick has. For people in larger bodies, an offset or swan-neck handle may be better as it distributes your weight evenly across the top of the stick. For people with wrist and hand weakness, a Fischer handle may be preferred, as it is ergonomically shaped to spread the weight evenly across the hand. Before purchasing a walking stick, research the different types and materials to ensure you are getting the correct one for your individual needs.

In my personal experience with mobility aids, I began by using my sister's crutches from a previous illness. Having these as a starting point allowed me to try out a mobility aid with no added expense. Once I began to see a benefit from using them, I knew I needed to invest in my own pair. I started out by purchasing a cheap folding walking stick from Amazon but as I am overweight, it was not well suited to me. While researching, I found that a swan-neck handle is best suited to overweight people and so I purchased one of these. I made sure that it is a height-adjustable one so I can wear different-height shoes. Mine is also made of aluminium, which means it is strong enough to hold my weight and use every day but also reasonably priced.

After around a year or so had gone by, during which I used my walking stick every day, I noticed a general decline in my health. This meant I was not able to go out often, walk for very long or carry heavy weights. At this point I decided to invest in a rollator. I chose this mobility aid because it offers two-handed support and a place to sit down when I become too tired. It also has storage space for any items I need to carry and adjustable-height arms. This checked all of the boxes, especially as it also has a very lightweight frame that I can easily lift, even without assistance, and a seat wide enough to fit me. Once I purchased my rollator I gained back some independence I thought I had lost forever. I am now able to go out for short walks whenever I want, and to go to the shops and bring items home in the storage bag under the seat. Having my rollator also means I always have a seat when I'm on public transport, which is helpful for getting to hospital and doctors' appointments.

Currently, I use my walking stick most days inside my home, or for short walks outside. I use my rollator for longer-distance walks outside, day trips out and going to any appointments or procedures. Using my mobility aids has changed the way I feel about my life (see figure 8, below) means I can go out and about with confidence and independence. I do not need to schedule my life around when a family member is available to drive me places and I can save money on cab fares by using public transport again.

Figure 8 How I feel when I use my mobility aids

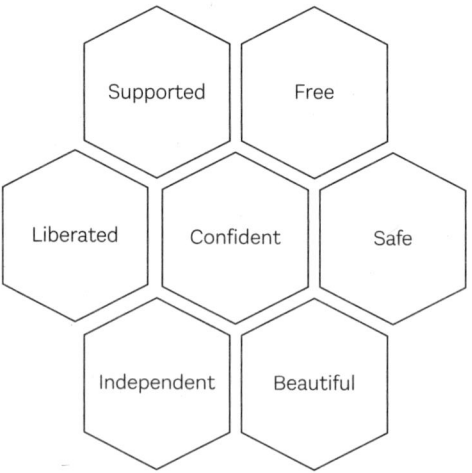

Community column

'I'm always worried that I don't actually need a mobility aid. I've wanted one since I was in kindergarten because of the pain, but my parents refused. They said wheelchairs were only for elderly people or those who can't walk. I had to wait until I was an adult to get one for myself, and I'm sure my parents disapprove.' – Mari

'I couldn't be without mine [mobility aid] now! Shopping without my scooter is impossible. I get stared at all the time or treated like I'm entirely invisible but whatever; they aren't people I would want to interact with anyway!' – Lucy

'I wish [people] understood that I don't always need mobility aids but sometimes I do. I want people to understand that mobility aids are freedom, not a downer.' – Bri

Reflections

Have you ever considered using a mobility aid?

Which one/s do you think you'd find beneficial?

If you already use a mobility aid, how has it impacted your life?

4

Hospital visits and medical admin

A big part of daily life with a chronic illness, condition and disability will involve both hospitals and medical admin, so this chapter is one you will likely need at some point, even if you haven't already. You may not need to stay in hospitals often, but it could be something that affects you in the future. For this reason you should consider in advance what may need to be packed into your hospital bag, whether for a planned procedure or in case of an emergency.

In addition, the importance of medical admin cannot be overstated. Keeping your records in order and easily accessible will save you time, spoons and stress and ensure you have to hand anything you may need in terms of paperwork and information about your medical history, medication and diagnoses.

What goes in my hospital bag?

If your illness is unstable enough that you may end up in the emergency department without warning, you may need to have a hospital bag permanently packed and ready to go at a moment's notice. You may also need to pack a hospital bag on a more ad hoc basis for planned procedures and treatments.

It can be overwhelming to put together a hospital bag, especially the first time, as it is difficult to know what you may need or how long your stay will be. If you are packing for a planned procedure or treatment then your medical care team or the doctor carrying out the procedure will usually be able to tell you how long you will be in hospital for, so don't be afraid to ask. If you are packing your hospital bag in case of an emergency, a good time frame to pack for is a week. Carers or loved ones can bring clean items if you are there for longer than that.

As well as what you do want to bring, think about what *not* to bring. I'd avoid any valuables (apart from your phone) that you wouldn't want to go missing, and be wary of having too much cash in your purse.

To make the packing process less daunting, I have made a detailed list of everything you may need to put in your bag:

1. Medical records
2. Clothing
3. Toiletries
4. Entertainment
5. Additional essentials

1. Medical records

- A copy of your medical summary (*see* p. 217 for tips on writing one)
- Photocopies of your medical diagnoses, with information of when you were diagnosed, where and by whom. Include information on your main symptoms and their severity if possible
- A list of your known allergies and intolerances as well as your dietary requirements (halal, gluten-free, etc.)
- Any aids you require, such as a wheelchair, rollator or crutches
- Emergency contact information for your next of kin, including their name, telephone number and relationship to you

2. Clothing

- Multiple sets of pyjamas or comfortable clothes you can wear while resting during your hospital stay

- Several days' worth of underwear, including non-slip socks if you have any
- Slippers or sliders to wear around the ward and into the bathrooms during your stay
- A set of comfortable clothes to wear home from the hospital, such as sweatpants, a hoodie and comfortable shoes

3. Toiletries

- Toothbrush and toothpaste
- Wash cloth and body wash or soap
- Dry shampoo
- Hand sanitiser
- Hair ties
- Period products
- Deodorant
- Earplugs
- Face wipes
- Eye mask
- Glasses and/or contact lens case

4. Entertainment

- Headphones for music, movies and phone calls
- Books to read
- Puzzle books (crosswords, wordsearch, sudoku, etc.)
- Phone, e-reader, tablet or other entertainment device
- Charger cables for all devices

5. Additional essentials

- Notepad and pen
- Non-perishable snacks, such as cereal bars or dried fruit
- Small amounts of cash or coins for buying food, drink and other items in the hospital
- A spare bag for dirty laundry
- Your regular medications you take on a daily basis

Things to remember
- Let your loved ones and carers know where your pre-packed hospital bag is, in case of emergency.
- Put your name and contact information on a label on your bag.
- Never take original copies of your records, only photocopies (as the hospital may need to keep them).
- Travel-sized toiletries are great for saving space in your bag.
- For longer hospital stays, a bath towel may be necessary for bathing. Hospitals provide these but you may be more comfortable with your own.
- Hospitals are usually not liable for theft and damage to your personal items, so be mindful when packing your expensive devices.
- Duffle bags or hand luggage bags with multiple pockets and compartments are excellent for staying organised, as are packing cubes.
- Keep records and medications in a separate, easily reachable compartment to ensure they are on hand immediately.
- Keep your records and medication list up to date at all times and available in your pre-packed bag.

Managing medications

Throughout this book we have discussed the importance of taking your medications at the correct times and dosages. Figuring this out can involve some trial and error, but having a routine you can stick to will go a long way in helping you to manage your chronic illness, condition or disability. Below are some helpful ways to ensure you are taking your medications correctly:

1. Pill boxes
2. Reminders
3. Paper tracking

1. Pill boxes

Having your medications organised into pill boxes is an excellent way to ensure you are taking the correct dosages at the right times. These pill boxes are widely available in shops, pharmacies or online and can be fairly cheap. When purchasing a medication organiser make sure it is suitable for your needs. If you only take medications once per day, a single-slot organiser will work. However, if you are taking medications multiple times per day, purchase an organiser with the correct amount of slots to make sure you are not skipping doses. In some pharmacies, Dosette boxes are made up by the pharmacist for people on stable and regular medications to ensure they are taken correctly. Speak to your doctor or pharmacist to see if this is suitable for you, or buy your own pill box and organise your medications for yourself.

2. Reminders

Setting reminders and alarms on your phone or another device is an excellent way to ensure you are taking your medications correctly and at the right times. Each alarm can be labelled differently and repeated regularly, meaning you just set them once and they repeat daily (or whenever you need them).

3. Paper tracking

Paper tracking involves physically writing out your medication dosages and using some kind of chart or grid to manually tick off when you have taken them. This is a good way for you or your carers to check in and see if and when medications have been taken and is especially useful for people who may not be able to remember if doses have been taken and want to see, at a glance, if they have. Table 10, on the next page, is an example of the type of grid that could be used to track your medication intake.

Table 10 Sample medication tracker

	Monday	Tuesday	Wednesday	Thursday	Friday	Saturday	Sunday
Morning							
Afternoon							
Evening							
Night							

A simple design such as this can be hand-drawn or created digitally and printed for use. It is easily customisable and can be adapted to meet your own needs. For example, the number of doses can be changed, and you could add a section for each individual medication or any medications that are taken less regularly, such as a weekly injection or transdermal patches.

As with most things on your spoonie journey, you need to find a system for managing medication that works for you. This may involve trial and error, including combining these tips and using more than one to keep you on track, or finding and creating your own system.

Filing your medical records

Organising your medical records at home can be a pain to do. Nobody warns you how much paperwork a chronic illness, condition or disability actually generates! If you're anything like me, you have countless letters from different doctors, in different specialities, summarising your conditions, your medications and lots of other things.

It is crucial that you effectively manage all of this paperwork, because if you have loose paper everywhere it can mean important documents get lost and appointments get missed.

Some services have apps where you can access your hospital letters, consultations and prescriptions digitally. This can help reduce the burden of paperwork (and save a few trees!), so do look into this if your care provider offers it as an option.

Personally, I have created a large, easily accessible folder where I keep all of my medical paperwork. To keep it organised, the folder is subdivided into six categories, each with a different wallet:

1. Medical summary
2. Essential medical letters
3. Medicine list
4. Hospital discharge papers
5. Non-essential medical letters
6. Letters from 'xyz' specialist

1. Medical summary

This should be in a plastic wallet at the very front of your folder and include all important information about your illness. A copy should also be kept in your hospital bag, if you have one. The summary does not need to be fancy or complicated: just create a simple document that can make it easier to provide a run-down of your medical history when you need to. This should include information such as:

1. Name, date of birth, address and contact information
2. You GP's name, address and contact information
3. You emergency contact's name and contact information
4. Your diagnoses (include where they were diagnosed and when)
5. Your current medications, doses and when taken
6. Treatments tried and when

2. Essential medical letters

This wallet includes medical letters that reference a specific diagnosis. These may need to be easily accessible in a rush and should include evidence of your diagnoses or treatments. Photocopies of these letters should be taken when you see a new doctor or specialist, so they can see evidence of your previous diagnoses.

3. Medicine list

Your medicine list is a list of your current medications and their dosages and side effects. This also includes a list of medications you have tried in the past to manage your symptoms, any side effects and when you tried them. Try to be as accurate as possible to ensure clarity.

4. Hospital discharge letters

If you are admitted to the hospital for any reason, including emergencies and planned procedures, you are usually given discharge papers explaining the reason for your stay, the treatment and medications given. These letters should all be kept together in a wallet in case you need them in the future. I personally prefer to keep them in chronological order for clarity and convenience.

5. Non-essential medical letters

This file should contain any letters from your medical care team that are non-critical, but that you still need to keep hold of. For example, I have endless appointments where doctors attempt to adjust my medications in tiny increments. After each of these tweaks I get a letter explaining what happened during the appointment. These letters are not exactly essential, but it is still a good idea to keep them for at least one or two years.

6. Letters from 'xyz' specialist

These are letters from individual specialists. They usually contain a quick summary of everything discussed during your appointment with that doctor, any planned treatments, and changes to medications. Keeping each specialist in a separate folder can make accessing information at a later date much easier.

Conclusion

I sincerely hope that you have found some helpful advice and management techniques among the pages of this book. The main reason I decided to write it was to help people like you survive your day-to-day life with a chronic illness, condition or disability. I know I keep saying it, but to reiterate the main message I want to convey: pacing and conserving your spoons really are essential. Prioritising your own needs and desires should also be non-negotiable and advocating for yourself is a major and unavoidable part of life with a chronic illness.

A huge part of managing your spoonie life successfully comes from accurately assessing your own needs. This is something that will take time and practice to learn and get right. I won't sugarcoat it: you will get it wrong a lot of the time. You will overestimate your abilities or underestimate how much rest you need. What is important is that you learn from these mistakes and implement what you have learned in your daily life, wherever necessary. Use those lessons to do better next time and the next time and the next time.

I invite you now to take the important step of really making time to explore and discover your own needs and limitations. Use this book as a jumping-off point, implement the strategies and tips I have outlined here and adapt them to your own needs. Remember, there is no single chronic illness or disabled experience. The information in this book is an amalgamation of hacks and tips I have found helpful in my own life, as well as those shared by thousands of online spoonies. Some of it may not apply to you; some of it may be ill-suited to your own life; some of it may not be relevant right now but it could be one day. Learning to adapt and change to better suit your own needs is an essential skill when you have an illness that is constantly changing and adapting, too. Use those skills to create the type of life you want.

Your old life and the life you thought you would have are gone. So now you have to create the kind of life you want to have, in the circumstances you are living with. Just because your life looks different now, it does not mean it is not a good life. Find pockets of peace and moments of beauty in the mundane and enjoy what you've got. Be proud of who you are and look forward to who you will become.

If I could give you one final piece of advice it would be this: share this book with all those around you: your friends and family and your carers. I say this not to sell more books but so that others can begin to understand what your life is like. I want everyone to acknowledge how difficult it is to live with a chronic illness, condition or disability. I would like you to be able to discuss your needs and wants with them, for them to understand all of the things you go through that they have the privilege of not needing to think about. I want you to share this book with them so you can learn more about each other.

Share this book with them so that *you are not alone.*

Acknowledgements

First and foremost, I want to thank my parents, Kay and Avtar, for their ongoing and total support throughout this process. You both encouraged me to embark upon this journey and without you both there would be no book at all.

Mum, you were right. You believed I could write a book and now thanks to your constant encouragement (read: hounding) and your belief in my abilities, I've managed it. Thank you for keeping me on track and feel free to say, 'I told you so.'

Dad, your quiet words of encouragement and advice have kept me sane and helped me keep perspective. Through all of the anxiety you've kept me level and kept me from spiralling, probably more times than you realise. Thank you for always being the calm in the storm.

I also want to thank and acknowledge my siblings. Sandy and Belinda, you have always and will always keep me going and keep me smiling. Your constant bickering in the background made for excellent white noise so I could lock in and meet my deadlines. Sophie, your presence and advice throughout this whole long process has been invaluable and I appreciated having a place to turn whenever I needed it.

Massi, you have always been a continual source of support, guidance and comfort all throughout my chronic illness journey. You've encouraged my work online and shown me that living well with chronic pain is absolutely possible. You've proven that you can live with an illness and still keep doing what you love and shining bright. You are an inspiration to me always and this book is for you more than anybody else.

I would also like to thank my friends, Kam and Anisha, for all of your advice and guidance throughout. Having you both to turn to when I'm stuck or need an opinion has been so important in getting this book finished. Thank you for hyping me up, letting me bounce around ideas and constantly encouraging me since we met all those years ago. I'm grateful to you both for everything you have done and continue to do for me.

I would also like to acknowledge all of those people who have interacted with my content online because you have helped me bring this book to life. Every like, comment and share has contributed to this book in a real and tangible way, because without them, it would never have been written. A few quick clicks from you all over the years have forever changed my life and I'll never stop being grateful.

I want to give a final thank you to everyone at Bloomsbury Publishing for making this book a reality. The editorial team, particularly Holly and Megan, have assisted in every way possible, have ensured this whole process has been smooth sailing and that my needs have been taken into account the entire way. I could not have asked for a more caring and considerate team of dedicated and amazing people to work with, and I look forward to seeing what we can come up with next.

References

Introduction

The 'spoon theory'... created in 2003 by Christine Miserandino: Latifi, F., 'Spoon theory: What it is and how I use it to manage chronic illness', *The Washington Post*, 14 January 2023: https://www.washingtonpost.com/wellness/2023/01/14/spoon-theory-chronic-illness-spoonie/

Part 1, chapter 2

Managing chronic pain: Foster, M., 'Pathways through persistent pain: Tips for managing chronic pain', Mayo Clinic Health System, 26 May 2023: https://www.mayoclinichealthsystem.org/hometown-health/speaking-of-health/8-tips-for-managing-chronic-pain

Something as minor as a common cold or flu: Black, R., 'Getting a Cold or the Flu When You Already Have Chronic Pain', HealthCentral, 28 January 2019: https://www.healthcentral.com/condition/infectious-disease/getting-cold-flu-when-you-already-have-chronic-pain

Around 5.8 per cent of the global population used drugs at least once in 2021: 'Opioid overdose', World Health Organization, 29 August 2023: https://www.who.int/news-room/fact-sheets/detail/opioid-overdose.

Signs of narcotic addiction: 'Opioid medicines and the risk of addiction', Medicines and Healthcare products Regulatory Agency, 23 September 2020: https://www.gov.uk/guidance/narcotic-medicines-and-the-risk-of-addiction

Experiencing withdrawal effects when you stop taking them [narcotics]: Case-Lo, C., 'Withdrawing from Opiates and Opioids', Healthline, 13 December 2024: https://www.healthline.com/health/opiate-withdrawal#symptoms

Part 1, chapter 3

The causes of fatigue usually fit into one of three main categories: Marcin, A., 'Causes of Fatigue and How to Manage It', *Healthline*, 23 May 2018: https://www.healthline.com/health/fatigue#causes

Part 2, chapter 1

Mental health conditions are much more likely: 'Long-term physical conditions and mental health', Mental Health Foundation, 18 February 2022: https://www.mentalhealth.org.uk/explore-mental-health/a-z-topics/long-term-physical-conditions-and-mental-health.

The link between chronic illness and mental health: Huang, Y., Loux, T., Huang, X. and Feng, X., 'The relationship between chronic diseases and mental health: A cross-sectional study', *Mental Health & Prevention* (32), December 2023: https://www.sciencedirect.com/science/article/abs/pii/S2212657023000491

Symptoms of depression: 'Signs you may be struggling to cope', The Samaritans: https://www.samaritans.org/how-we-can-help/if-youre-having-difficult-time/signs-you-may-be-struggling-cope/

Experiencing symptoms of depression for extended periods of time: 'Treatment – Depression in adults', NHS, 5 July 2023: https://www.nhs.uk/mental-health/conditions/depression-in-adults/treatment/

There are many different types of depression: 'Types of Depression', Mental Health UK: https://mentalhealth-uk.org/help-and-information/conditions/depression/types-of-depression/

Generalised anxiety disorder: 'Generalised anxiety disorder (GAD)', NHS, 22 October 2021: https://www.nhs.uk/mental-health/conditions/generalised-anxiety-disorder-gad.

Social anxiety: 'Social anxiety (social phobia)', NHS, 17 May 2023: https://www.nhs.uk/mental-health/conditions/social-anxiety/

Health anxiety: 'Health anxiety', NHS, 8 November 2023: https://www.nhs.uk/mental-health/conditions/health-anxiety/

Part 2, chapter 2

Medical gaslighting is unfortunately a common occurrence: Vinney, C., 'How to Spot Medical Gaslighting and What to Do About It', VeryWellMind, 18 May 2023: https://www.verywellmind.com/what-is-medical-gaslighting-6831284

There is a distinct lack of medical data in female bodies: Balch, B., 'Why we know so little about women's health', AAMC, March 2024: https://www.aamc.org/news/why-we-know-so-little-about-women-s-health

A survey in 2019: 'Feel discriminated against at the doctor's office? TODAY survey finds you're not alone', TODAY, May 2019: https://www.today.com/health/today-survey-finds-gender-discrimination-doctor-s-office-serious-issue-t153641

A study of 4700 medical students: Phelan, S. M., Dovidio, J. F., Puhl, R. M., Burgess, D. J., Nelson, D. B., Yeazel, M. W., Hardeman, R., Perry, S. and van Ryn, M., 'Implicit and explicit weight bias in a national sample of 4,732 medical students: The medical student CHANGES study', Obesity (22): 1201–1208, 2014: https://onlinelibrary.wiley.com/doi/10.1002/oby.20687

In 2016 a study found that nearly half: Sabin, J., 'How we fail black patients in pain', AAMC, January 2020: https://www.aamc.org/news/how-we-fail-black-patients-pain

Part 2, chapter 4

Imposter syndrome... can be experienced in all areas of life: Cuncic, A., 'Is Imposter Syndrome Holding You Back From Living Your Best Life', Verywell Mind, September 2024: https://www.verywellmind.com/imposter-syndrome-and-social-anxiety-disorder-4156469

Imposter syndrome is common and **Invisible illnesses:** Wiesmann, T., 'From Self-Doubt to Self-Assurance: Navigating Imposter Syndrome in Chronic Illness', Hypermobility MD, January 2024: https://www.hypermobilitymd.com/post/from-self-doubt-to-self-assurance-navigating-imposter-syndrome-in-chronic-illness.

Experience of being medically gaslit by healthcare professionals: Geraghty, M., 'Imposter Syndrome in Migraine and Chronic Pain', National Headache Foundation, September 2024: https://headaches.org/imposter-syndrome-in-migraine-and-chronic-pain/

Experience of being medically gaslit by loved ones: Jordan, E., 'Am I sick enough? Living with Imposter Syndrome', Crohn's & Colitis UK, 30 October 2019: https://crohnsandcolitis.org.uk/news-stories/blog-posts/am-i-an-impostor

Part 2, chapter 5

Signs of burnout: 'Burnout', Mental Health UK: https://mentalhealth-uk.org/burnout/#section-3

Types of boundaries and what they mean: Earnshaw, E., '6 Types Of Boundaries You Deserve To Have (And How To Maintain Them)', MindBodyGreen, December 2022: https://www.mindbodygreen.com/articles/six-types-of-boundaries-and-what-healthy-boundaries-look-like-for-each

Part 3, chapter 1

Have far fewer usable hours in a day: Garlit, D., 'How Much Usable Time Do We Have?', Multiplesclerosis.net, June 2022: https://multiplesclerosis.net/living-with-ms/productivity

Part 3, chapter 2

There is a huge variety of hidden and additional costs: Elizabeth, L., 'The Cost of Comfort with Chronic Illness', The Century Foundation, May 2023: https://tcf.org/content/commentary/the-cost-of-comfort-with-chronic-illness/ and Wright, S., Field, S., Moss, C., Frounks, A. and Veruete-McKay, L., 'Disability Price Tag 2024', Scope, September 2024: https://www.scope.org.uk/campaigns/disability-price-tag

Part 3, chapter 3

The three key approaches listed below: Foxwell, A., 'Accessibility In Education: 5 Ways to Help', ReadSpeaker, June 2022: https://www.readspeaker.com/blog/education-accessibility/

To allow them to remain in school: Downey, C., '6 Ways To Make Learning Accessible To All Students', Rev, February 2022: https://www.rev.com/blog/speech-to-text-accessibility/6-ways-to-make-learning-accessible-to-all-students

These different learning styles include: 'What are the 7 different learning styles and do they work?', Avado, July 2021: https://www.avadolearning.com/blog/the-7-different-learning-styles-and-what-they-mean/

Students taking exams throughout the year: 'What are exam access arrangements?', Everway: https://www.texthelp.com/en-gb/resources/inclusive-education/access-arrangements/

Access needs can include adjustments: 'Accessibility at work', ACAS, November 2024: https://www.acas.org.uk/accessibility-at-work

Part 3, chapter 4

Selling fake or misleading products and **things that mark out a health and well-being scam:** 'Common Health Scams', Federal Trade Commission Consumer Advice, October 2024: https://consumer.ftc.gov/articles/common-health-scams

Helpful resources

Four More Spoons Instagram Account (Jodie K Ranu)
www.instagram.com/fourmorespoons

Befrienders Worldwide (Global Suicide Prevention) – Search for your local mental health hotline by country
befrienders.org/

NHS Website – For accurate information about conditions, symptoms and tests
www.nhs.uk/health-a-to-z/

Mayo Clinic Website – For accurate information about conditions and illnesses
www.mayoclinic.org/

Index

access 180
    advocating for 154–5
    to education 149–52
    in the workplace 152–4
acute pain 39, 41, 47
addiction
    to narcotics 55–6
    treatment scams 161
advocating
    for accessibility 154–5
    for yourself in the health sector 8–9, 91, 96–101
alarms/reminders, setting 30
anti-ageing products 160
anxiety 21, 82, 95, 122
    generalised anxiety disorder (GAD) 82–3
    health 85–8
    social 84–5
    treatments 81, 83, 85, 87
appointments, medical
    advocating for yourself 8–9, 91, 96–101
    hospital visits - points to remember 214
    medical gaslighting 37, 49, 89–94, 116, 117
    packing your hospital bag 211–13
    preparation and symptom tracking 33–8, 96–101, 119
arthritis treatment scams 161

baseline symptoms *v* flare-ups 13–14
boom-bust cycle 72–3
boundaries 8, 66, 126–9
    how to implement 129–31
brain fog 27–30, 31, 79, 123
burnout
    managing 123–6
    setting boundaries 126–31
    signs of 121–3

cancer cure scams 159–60
carers *see* support
Chronic Fatigue Syndrome (CFS) 140

chronic pain 40
    cycles 41–2
    impact of 43–4
    managing 45–6
    and narcotics 50–6
    pain scale 47–9
cleaning your home 183–8
    asking for help 191
    kitchen jobs 190–1
    knowing your limitations 191–2
    prioritising 185–6, 188–92
    recycling/general waste bins 186–7
    useful equipment 187–8
clothing 25, 180, 212–13
cognitive behaviour therapy (CBT) 81, 83, 85, 87
colds and flu, impact of 22, 45
comfort, your 25
cooking, preparing food and 19, 192–6
cost of spoonie living *see* finances

dehydration 19, 24, 125
delivery services and post 145, 197, 199–200, 201–2
depression 21, 78, 95, 122, 170
    symptoms 78–9
    treatment options 81
    types of 79–81
diabetes 18, 140, 160
diagnosis, not having a 116, 118
dynamic disabilities 116, 117

education accessibility 149–52
employment 135–7
    accessibility in the workplace 152–4

errands, running 197–202
exercise and movement 45–6

family and friends 23–4, 99–100, 119, 126, 136, 170–1
    unsupportive people 103–5, 117–18, 173
    see also support
fatigue 31, 57, 122–3
    causes of 57–9
    four Ps of fatigue management 59–60
finances
    hidden costs of spoonie life 143–8, 177
    loss of income 135–42
flare-ups 13–14, 15, 16, 115, 117
    common causes 16–22
    common ways to manage 22–5
    and negative thoughts 26–7
food and drink 18–19, 24, 28, 79, 125, 145, 180
    preparing and cooking 192–6

gaslighting, medical 37, 49, 89–96, 116, 117
    self-gaslighting 95–6
going out 175–81

hospital bag, packing a 211–13

imposter syndrome and self-doubt 115–16
    ways to fight 118–20
    who might experience? 116–18
    see also gaslighting, medical
insomnia
    see sleep quality

invisible symptoms 31–3, 116
isolation 123, 147, 169–70
    see also social life; support

medical professionals 8–9, 124, 159, 165
    advocating for yourself 96–101
    changing your 100
    gaslighting 37, 49, 89–96, 116, 117
medical records, managing your 212, 216–18
medications
    access to your prescribed 198–200
    alternative remedies 146
    for anxiety and depression 81, 83, 85, 87
    costs 144
    and flare-ups 20
    health scams 157–65
    managing chronic pain 45, 50–6
    managing your 214–16
    missing/skipping 20–1
    painkillers and narcotics 24, 50–6, 78, 179
    prescription v non-prescription treatments 159
    travel plans 179
mental health 9, 57, 77, 147
    anxiety 82–8, 122
    depression 21, 78–82, 122
mindfulness and meditation 87
mobility aids/specialist equipment 144–5, 180, 203–5, 209
    choosing the right 205–8
    see also access
monitors, wearable 38

mood swings 122
multitasking 29

narcotics 50–2, 53–4, 78, 179
    addiction 55–6
    side-effects 52
    withdrawal symptoms 56
negative thoughts 26–7
    see also mental health
neurodivergent people 48, 49, 84
nutrition/diet 18–19, 24, 125, 145, 180, 192–6

online support and community 108–13
opiates and opioids *see* narcotics
overexertion 17–18, 23
overload, sensory 22
overweight/obesity, being 93

pacing yourself 8, 28, 46, 61, 63–4
    assessing whether to rest or participate 68–71
    boom-bust cycle 72–3
    how to successfully rest and pace 64–7
pain, living with
    acute pain 39, 41, 47
    chronic pain 40, 41–5, 48–9, 50–6
    medications/narcotics 24, 50–6
    treatment scams 160
pain scale 46–9
pill fatigue 20–1
plans, postponing/cancelling 24–5, 69–70, 173
prioritising activities and chores 65, 69–70, 185–6, 188–9

racial discrimination 93–4
rest 8, 23, 28, 64
   assessing whether to rest or participate 68–71
   boom-bust cycle 72–3
   boundary setting 66
   listening to your body 66
   prioritising activities 65
   recovery time 71
   scheduling rest days 64–5, 178–9
   screen time 66

scams, health/well-being 157–61
   how to avoid 164–5
   how to spot 161–3
screen time 18, 66
self-care, prioritising 8, 120, 125
self-doubt
   see imposter syndrome and self-doubt
self-harm and suicide 78
sensory issues 22, 31
sex 79, 128
sexual discrimination 92–3
shopping
   grocery 197–8
   non-grocery 200–1
sleep quality 18, 28, 46, 122, 125
social life
   loss of relationships 171–4
   planning ahead 175–81
   social withdrawal and isolation 123, 147, 169–70
   socialise the spoonie way 170–1
social media/online communities 108–13
spoon theory 5–7

stress 21, 28, 121, 123, 124
   see also burnout; mental health
support 119
   creating a spoonie community online 109–13
   financial 147
   finding community/networks 105–13, 123
   household chores 191
   lack of/unsupportive people 103–5, 117–18, 173
   online 108–13
   outsourcing tasks 126
   services 23–4, 46
symptoms
   baseline 13–15, 21
   diary keeping 886–87
   invisible 30–3
   management 9, 14–15, 22–30, 45–6
   tracking and analysing 33–8, 86–7, 119

to-do lists/planners 29–30, 60–1, 65–6, 188–9
tracking and analysing symptoms 33–8, 86–7, 119
travel/transport issues 145, 177–81

usable hours 137–9
   calculating your 139–41

vitamin and supplement scams 161

weather conditions 19–20, 81
weight biases 93
work–life balance 124

yourself, being 9